Essentials in Ophthalmology

Series Editor

Arun D. Singh

More information about this series at http://www.springer.com/series/5332

Rohit Varma • Benjamin Y. Xu
Grace M. Richter • Alena Reznik
Editors

Advances in Ocular Imaging in Glaucoma

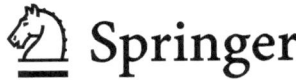

Springer

Editors
Rohit Varma, MD, MPH
Southern California Eye Institute
CHA Hollywood Presbyterian Medical
Center
Los Angeles, CA
USA

Benjamin Y. Xu, MD, PhD
Keck School of Medicine of USC
University of Southern California
Los Angeles, CA
USA

Grace M. Richter, MD, MPH
Keck School of Medicine of USC
University of Southern California
Los Angeles, CA
USA

Alena Reznik, MD
Southern California Eye Institute
CHA Hollywood Presbyterian Medical
Center
Los Angeles, CA
USA

ISSN 1612-3212   ISSN 2196-890X   (electronic)
Essentials in Ophthalmology
ISBN 978-3-030-43849-4   ISBN 978-3-030-43847-0   (eBook)
https://doi.org/10.1007/978-3-030-43847-0

© Springer Nature Switzerland AG 2020, corrected publication 2020
This work is subject to copyright. All rights are reserved by the Publisher, whether the whole or part of the material is concerned, specifically the rights of translation, reprinting, reuse of illustrations, recitation, broadcasting, reproduction on microfilms or in any other physical way, and transmission or information storage and retrieval, electronic adaptation, computer software, or by similar or dissimilar methodology now known or hereafter developed.
The use of general descriptive names, registered names, trademarks, service marks, etc. in this publication does not imply, even in the absence of a specific statement, that such names are exempt from the relevant protective laws and regulations and therefore free for general use.
The publisher, the authors, and the editors are safe to assume that the advice and information in this book are believed to be true and accurate at the date of publication. Neither the publisher nor the authors or the editors give a warranty, expressed or implied, with respect to the material contained herein or for any errors or omissions that may have been made. The publisher remains neutral with regard to jurisdictional claims in published maps and institutional affiliations.

This Springer imprint is published by the registered company Springer Nature Switzerland AG
The registered company address is: Gewerbestrasse 11, 6330 Cham, Switzerland

Preface

Traditionally, a glaucoma specialist simply performed gonioscopy, funduscopic optic disc examination, and visual field testing to diagnose and monitor disease progression. However, imaging technology from ultrasonography to optical coherence tomography (OCT) and beyond has demonstrated the vital role of such technological advancements in providing the best possible care for our glaucoma patients. The masses of literature to date in each area of glaucoma imaging technology can be overwhelming to even a glaucoma subspecialist. This book aims to serve as a primer on best practices for clinical integration of imaging technologies, interpretation of imaging, and a review of the clinically relevant literature of each technology. Furthermore, we offer an overview on new technological applications such as machine learning and retinal metabolic imaging, which are likely to become relevant to the glaucoma subspecialist's daily practice in the future. It is our hope that this book is valuable to ophthalmologists in training, comprehensive ophthalmologists, and glaucoma subspecialists alike.

Los Angeles, CA, USA

Rohit Varma
Benjamin Y. Xu
Grace M. Richter
Alena Reznik

The original version of this book was revised. Affiliation of book editor has been updated. A correction to this book can be found at https://doi.org/10.1007/978-3-030-43847-0_9

Contents

Contributors

Tin Aung, FRCSEd, PhD Singapore Eye Research Institute, Singapore National Eye Centre, Singapore, Singapore

Zhongping Chen, PhD Department of Biomedical Engineering and Beckman Laser Institute, University of California, Irvine, Irvine, CA, USA

Charles DeBoer, MD, PhD USC Roski Eye Institute, Keck Medicine of University of Southern California, Los Angeles, CA, USA

Department of Ophthalmology, LAC+USC Medical Center, Los Angeles, CA, USA

Jiun L. Do, MD, PhD Shiley Eye Institute, Department of Ophthalmology, University of California San Diego, La Jolla, CA, USA

Anthony E. Felder, PhD Richard & Loan Hill Department of Bioengineering, University of Illinois at Chicago, Chicago, IL, USA

Timothy P. Fox, MD Department of Ophthalmology, LAC+USC Medical Center, Los Angeles, CA, USA

Ahnul Ha, MD Department of Ophthalmology, Seoul National University College of Medicine, Seoul, Korea

Department of Ophthalmology, Seoul National University Hospital, Seoul, Korea

Mingguang He, MD, MPH, PhD Department of Ophthalmology, University of Melbourne, Centre for Eye Research Australia, East Melbourne, VIC, Australia

Youmin He, MS Department of Biomedical Engineering and Beckman Laser Institute, University of California, Irvine, Irvine, CA, USA

Hirut Kollech, MS, BS Computational Modeling and Simulation Program, Pittsburgh, PA, USA

Nils A. Loewen, MD, PhD, DMSc University of Würzburg, Department of Ophthalmology, Würzburg, Germany

Ralitsa T. Loewen, MD University of Pittsburgh, Department of Ophthalmology, Pittsburgh, PA, USA

Felipe Medeiros, MD, PhD Clinical Research Unit, Department of Ophthalmology, Duke University School of Medicine, Durham, NC, USA

Ki Ho Park, MD, PhD Department of Ophthalmology, Seoul National University College of Medicine, Seoul, Korea

Department of Ophthalmology, Seoul National University Hospital, Seoul, Korea

Yueqiao Qu, PhD Department of Biomedical Engineering and Beckman Laser Institute, University of California, Irvine, Irvine, CA, USA

Alena Reznik, MD Southern California Eye Institute, CHA Hollywood Presbyterian Medical Center, Los Angeles, CA, USA

Grace M. Richter, MD, MPH USC Roski Eye Institute, Keck Medicine of University of Southern California, Los Angeles, CA, USA

Mahnaz Shahidi, PhD USC Roski Eye Institute, Keck Medicine of University of Southern California, Los Angeles, CA, USA

Jing Shan, MD, PhD USC Roski Eye Institute, Keck Medicine of University of Southern California, Los Angeles, CA, USA

Department of Ophthalmology, LAC+USC Medical Center, Los Angeles, CA, USA

Jonathan Vande Geest, PhD Department of Bioengineering, University of Pittsburgh, Pittsburgh, PA, USA

Ruikang K. Wang, PhD University of Washington, Department of Bioengineering and Ophthalmology, Seattle, WA, USA

Susannah Waxman, BS University of Pittsburgh, School of Medicine, Interdisciplinary Biomedical Graduate Program, Pittsburgh, PA, USA

Brandon J. Wong, MD USC Roski Eye Institute, Keck Medicine of University of Southern California, Los Angeles, CA, USA

Benjamin Y. Xu, MD, PhD USC Roski Eye Institute, Keck Medicine of University of Southern California, Los Angeles, CA, USA

Department of Ophthalmology, Keck School of Medicine of University of Southern California, Los Angeles, CA, USA

Qifa Zhou, PhD Department of Ophthalmology, Keck School of Medicine of University of Southern California, Los Angeles, CA, USA

Department of Biomedical Engineering, University of Southern California, Los Angeles, CA, USA

Anterior Segment Optical Coherence Tomography

Benjamin Y. Xu, Jing Shan, Charles DeBoer, and Tin Aung

Introduction

Anterior segment optical coherence tomography (AS-OCT) is a relatively new in vivo imaging method that acquires cross-sectional images of the anterior segment and its structures by measuring their optical reflections [1]. AS-OCT devices have rapidly evolved over the past decade, integrating newer forms of OCT technology to improve imaging resolution and speed. Over that time, AS-OCT imaging has increased in popularity among clinicians and researchers, especially as a means of studying the anatomy and biomechanics of the anterior segment and its anatomical structures. However, there are few resources that teach the basics of qualitative and quantitative interpretation of AS-OCT images. This chapter acts as a guide for novice AS-OCT image graders while also providing the reader with information on OCT technology, clinical applications of AS-OCT imaging, and future directions of scientific research.

AS-OCT Technologies and Devices

AS-OCT imaging produces cross-sectional or volumetric scans of tissues in vivo or in vitro with micrometer resolution. Optical coherence tomography (OCT) technology is somewhat analogous to ultrasound technology, except that it utilizes light waves rather than sound waves to scan tissues. OCT technology relies on the principle of backscattered light, which is light that originates from a source and is reflected as it passes through materials or tissues. Backscattered light is detected by a sensor, which compares it to a reference light beam. The delay between the two beams provides information about the optical properties of the imaged material or tissue and defines boundaries between nonhomogeneous structures. In the eye, OCT image resolution and depth of penetration vary based on source light intensity and attenuation by intervening tissue structures. There are three commer-

B. Y. Xu (✉)
USC Roski Eye Institute, Keck Medicine
of University of Southern California,
Los Angeles, CA, USA

Department of Ophthalmology, Keck School of
Medicine of University of Southern California,
Los Angeles, CA, USA
e-mail: benjamix@usc.edu

J. Shan · C. DeBoer
USC Roski Eye Institute, Keck Medicine
of University of Southern California, Los Angeles,
CA, USA

Department of Ophthalmology, LAC+USC
Medical Center, Los Angeles, CA, USA

T. Aung
Singapore Eye Research Institute, Singapore National
Eye Centre, Singapore, Singapore

© Springer Nature Switzerland AG 2020
R. Varma et al. (eds.), *Advances in Ocular Imaging in Glaucoma*, Essentials in Ophthalmology,
https://doi.org/10.1007/978-3-030-43847-0_1

cially available OCT technologies that have been applied to AS-OCT imaging: time-domain OCT and Fourier-domain OCT, which can be subdivided into spectral-domain OCT and swept-source OCT.

The earliest AS-OCT devices were based on time-domain OCT technology. Due to limitations in time-domain OCT technology, early AS-OCT devices such as the Zeiss Visante (Carl Zeiss Meditec, Dublin, CA) and Heidelberg SL-OCT (Heidelberg Engineering, Heidelberg, Germany) had to sacrifice acquisition speed for spatial resolution [2]. These devices also used longer, 1310 μm wavelength light in order to increase imaging depth. As a result, images tended to be noisy and fine details of ocular structures, such as the trabecular meshwork, could not be resolved. In addition, the majority of early AS-OCT studies of the anterior segment were limited to a single cross-sectional OCT image acquired along the horizontal, temporal-nasal meridian. Finally, studies of early time-domain OCT devices reported poorer reliability and reproducibility compared to modern Fourier-domain OCT devices [3–8].

Fourier-domain OCT provides improvements in image quality and acquisition speed compared to time-domain OCT. Spectral-domain OCT devices such as the Zeiss Cirrus (Carl Zeiss Meditec, Dublin, CA) and Heidelberg Spectralis (Heidelberg Engineering, Heidelberg, Germany) utilize shorter wavelength light to produce images with enhanced spatial resolution, although this comes at the cost of imaging depth. This improvement enables more consistent visualization of Schlemm's canal and distal aqueous outflow structures on AS-OCT images. However, both devices require specialized lenses to acquire images that span the width of the anterior chamber. The Tomey CASIA SS-1000 (Tomey Corporation, Nagoya, Japan) is a swept-source Fourier-domain AS-OCT device that can acquire up to 128 cross-sectional OCT images in less than 2 seconds. However, due to its longer 1310 μm wavelength, its spatial resolution lags behind spectral-domain devices. Due to an overall increase in AS-OCT imaging speed,

the convention has shifted toward acquiring an increased number of images per eye. This change in methodology has been shown to increase the accuracy of AS-OCT imaging in terms of capturing anatomical variations inherent to the angle [9, 10].

Fourier-domain AS-OCT devices demonstrate excellent intra-examiner and inter-examiner reproducibility of measurements based on the location of the scleral spur or Schwalbe's line [11–15]. However, the correlation between measurements obtained on different devices varies depending on the parameter, ranging from poor to excellent [12, 14]. This difference likely arises from how different devices account for corneal refraction, which is a parameter used to scale and dewarp the corresponding OCT B-scans. Therefore, AS-OCT measurements should not be directly compared or used interchangeably between different devices.

The Iridocorneal Angle: Role in Aqueous Outflow and Assessment Methods

The irideocorneal angle is a key component of the conventional aqueous outflow pathway and plays a crucial role in the development of elevated intraocular pressure (IOP) and glaucomatous optic neuropathy. Aqueous humor is produced by the ciliary body and secreted into the posterior chamber (Fig. 1.1). From the posterior chamber, the aqueous humor flows through the iridolenticular junction, around the iris sphincter, and into the anterior chamber. From there it must pass through the iridocorneal angle to gain access the trabecular meshwork and distal outflow structures. The configuration of the iridocorneal angle and its constituent structures plays an important role in facilitating or impeding the flow of aqueous along this pathway. Appositional contact between the iris and trabecular meshwork can inhibit normal aqueous outflow, thereby leading to elevations of IOP, an important risk factor for the development of glaucomatous optic neuropathy.

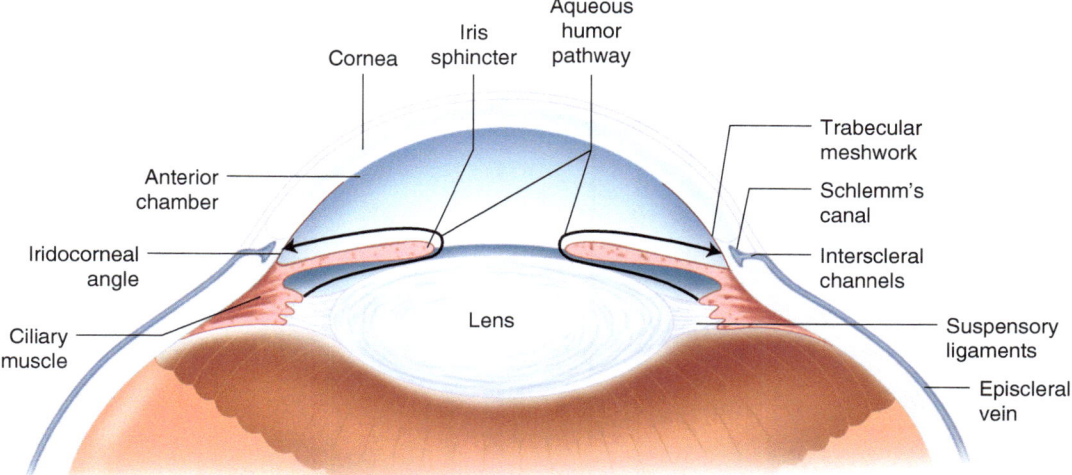

Fig. 1.1 Cross-sectional diagram of the anterior segment. Black arrows indicates the conventional aqueous outflow pathway from the ciliary muscle, around the iris sphincter, into the anterior chamber, and through the iridocorneal angle, trabecular meshwork, Schlemm's canal, interscleral (collector) channel, aqueous vein, and episcleral vein. Red line indicates the iridocorneal angle formed by anterior iris and posterior corneoscleral surfaces

AS-OCT imaging has modernized examination of the anterior segment, including the iridocorneal angle. However, to understand the clinical utility of AS-OCT imaging in glaucoma, it is necessary to discuss gonioscopy and ultrasound biomicroscopy (UBM), two angle assessment methods that preceded AS-OCT.

Gonioscopy is the current clinical standard for evaluating the iridocorneal angle (Fig. 1.2). Gonioscopy is a contact assessment method and requires that a specialized lens be placed on the corneal surface. The goniolens permits a view of the iridocorneal angle either through direct examination, in the case of a direct goniolens (e.g., Koeppe), or indirect examination through a mirror, in the case of indirect goniolenses (e.g., Posner-Zeiss, Goldmann). Indirect gonioscopy is typically preferred over direct gonioscopy since it can be performed with the patient seated at a slit lamp, which increases viewing stability and allows for image magnification. Gonioscopy is also the current clinical standard for detecting angle closure, defined as inability to visualize the pigmented trabecular meshwork, and primary angle closure disease (PACD), defined as gonioscopic angle closure in three or more angle quadrants [16].

Gonioscopy has several limitations despite being the current clinical standard. Gonioscopy is a subjective assessment method requiring considerable examiner expertise. Special attention must be paid to ensure the slit beam does not cross the pupillary margin, which can cause pupillary constriction and widening of the iridocorneal angle. Indentation of the cornea by the goniolens can also induce angle widening or corneal striae, both of which affect the visibility of angle structures. Gonioscopy is also associated with high interobserver variability, even among experienced glaucoma specialists [17]. These differences may be related to patient eye deviations or degree of lens tilting by the examiner, which are aspects of gonioscopy that are difficult to quantify or standardize across examinations. Finally, gonioscopy is a qualitative assessment method. While numerical grades are often assigned to angle quadrants based on identification of anatomical landmarks, these numbers are subjective and categorical in nature. Therefore, there are limited clinical methods based on gonioscopy to track progression of

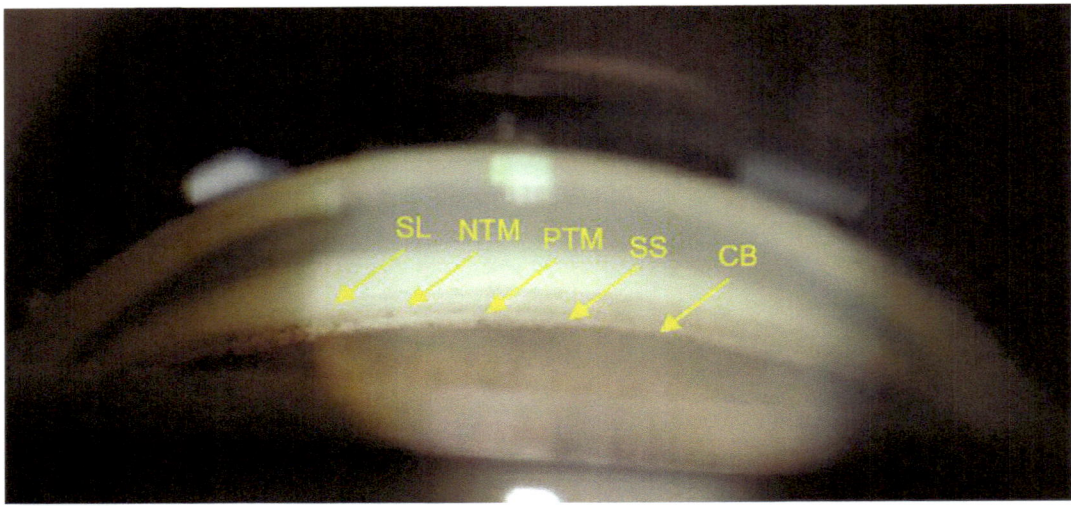

Fig. 1.2 A gonioscopic view of an open iridocorneal angle. Arrows indicate Schwalbe's line (SL), non-pigmented trabecular meshwork (NTM), pigmented trabecular meshwork (PTM), scleral spur (SS), and ciliary body (CB)

angle closure over time or assess patient response to interventions intended to alleviate angle closure, such as LPI.

UBM is an alternative method to assess the anterior segment and its structures. UBM utilizes sound waves that are shorter in wavelength than those used in conventional ocular ultrasonography, which provides increased spatial resolution at the cost of reduced depth of penetration through the sclera. UBM provides qualitative and quantitative assessments of the anterior segment, including the posterior chamber the ciliary body. However, studies demonstrate variable reproducibility of quantitative measurements of anterior chamber parameters, including those that quantify angle width [18, 19]. UBM is also a contact assessment method requiring a trained, experienced examiner. Therefore, its use is limited primarily to glaucoma practices or tertiary referral centers.

AS-OCT provides several advantages over gonioscopy. AS-OCT imaging does not require contact, thus minimizing test-induced distortions of angle configuration. Nor does it require an experienced examiner, as AS-OCT imaging can be performed by a technician with a limited amount of training. AS-OCT imaging also provides quantitative measurements of the anterior

segment and its structures, including the width of the iridocorneal angle. Gonioscopy also provides several advantages over AS-OCT. Gonioscopy can be performed with a goniolens at a slit lamp and does not require expensive, specialized equipment. Certain qualitative exam findings, such as peripheral anterior synechiae (PAS) or neovascularization of the angle (NVA), are easier to detect on gonioscopy than AS-OCT. Finally, the clinical relevance of gonioscopy is well supported by a robust body of literature that defines its role in the detection and management of PACD.

AS-OCT imaging resembles UBM imaging in that both provide qualitative and quantitative assessments of the anterior segment. However, AS-OCT provides several advantages over UBM. One advantage is improved spatial resolution, which allows for more reliable detection of key anatomical landmarks, such as the scleral spur. Another advantage is faster imaging speed since AS-OCT does not require probe movements to image different portions of the angle. A third advantage is its noncontact nature; in the absence of a probe applied to the ocular surface, the subject can fixate on a visual stimulus, thereby stabilizing the eye. The combined effect of these two factors is an increase in inter-observer reproducibility, especially among modern Fourier-domain

OCT devices [3–8]. The primary shortcoming of AS-OCT compared to UBM is its inability to visualize anatomical structures posterior to the iris, including the ciliary body. This limits the utility of AS-OCT in diagnosing certain causes of angle closure, such as plateau iris syndrome and iris or ciliary body neoplasms.

Aqueous Outflow Pathways

AS-OCT imaging has been applied to the study of conventional and nonconventional aqueous outflow pathways. The trabecular meshwork and Schlemm's canal are more easily visible on shorter wavelength spectral-domain OCT devices, such as Cirrus and Spectralis (Fig. 1.3), compared to longer wavelength AS-OCT devices, such as CASIA. These devices permit in vivo 360-degree visualization of the proximal structures of the conventional aqueous outflow pathway [20]. Distal aqueous outflow structures, such as collector channels and aqueous veins, are visible on longer wavelength experimental Fourier-domain AS-OCT devices designed to penetrate through the scleral wall [21–23]. The suprachoroidal component of the nonconventional outflow pathway is visible when there is increased fluid in the space, as in the case of uveal effusion or after glaucoma surgery [24–26].

AS-OCT studies of the conventional aqueous outflow pathway have shed light on possible mechanisms by which medications and surgery lower IOP. For example, in vivo AS-OCT imaging has been used to confirm that pilocarpine increases the lumen size of Schlemm's canal in eyes with and without glaucoma [9]. Dilations of Schlemm's canal are also observable after phacoemulsification surgery, and the magnitudes of dilation are correlated with decreases in IOP [27].

Interpretation of AS-OCT Images

AS-OCT images can be interpreted qualitatively, similar to slit lamp assessments of the anterior chamber and gonioscopic assessments of the iridocorneal angle. Some key structures, such as the cornea, lens, and iris, are easily identifiable in AS-OCT images, even to a novice examiner (Fig. 1.4). However, examining the iridotrabecular angle, formed by the junction between the trabecular meshwork and anterior iris surface, for evidence of angle closure is not as intuitive. The imaging-based definition of angle closure is iridotrabecular contact, which is apposition between the trabecular meshwork and anterior surface of the iris (Fig. 1.5). The visibility of the trabecular meshwork on AS-OCT is dependent on a number of factors, including eye stability and quality of the ocular surface. The trabecular meshwork is also easier to visualize on devices utilizing newer OCT technologies or shorter wavelengths of light, such as the Zeiss Cirrus and Heidelberg Spectralis (Fig. 1.3). However, visualizing the trabecular meshwork, Schlemm's canal, and distal outflow pathways is not necessary to identify appositional angle closure.

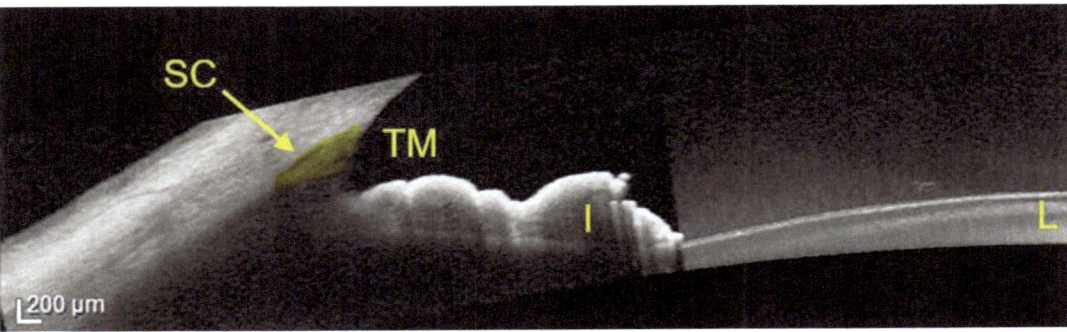

Fig. 1.3 Image taken with the Heidelberg Spectralis with anterior segment module. The iris (I), lens (L), trabecular meshwork (TM), and Schlemm's canal (SC, yellow arrow) are marked

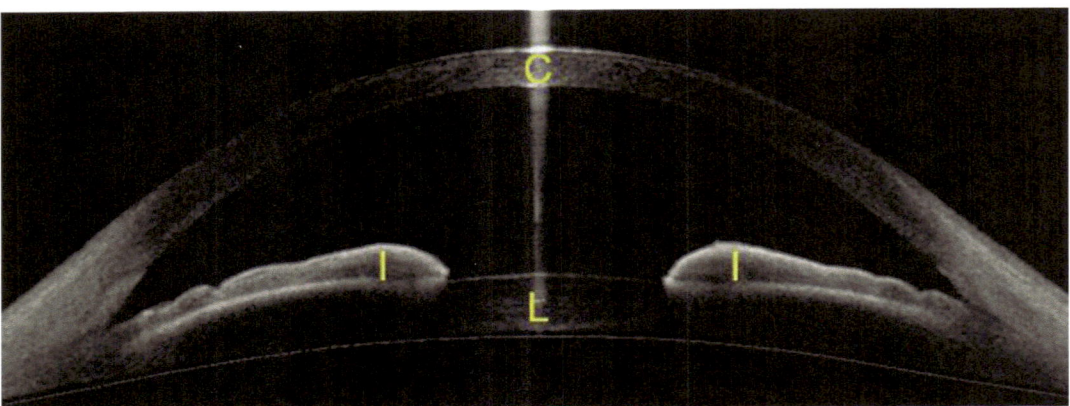

Fig. 1.4 Image taken with the Tomey CASIA SS-1000 demonstrating typical cross-sectional view of the anterior segment along the horizontal, temporal-nasal meridian. The cornea (C), iris (I), and lens (L) are marked

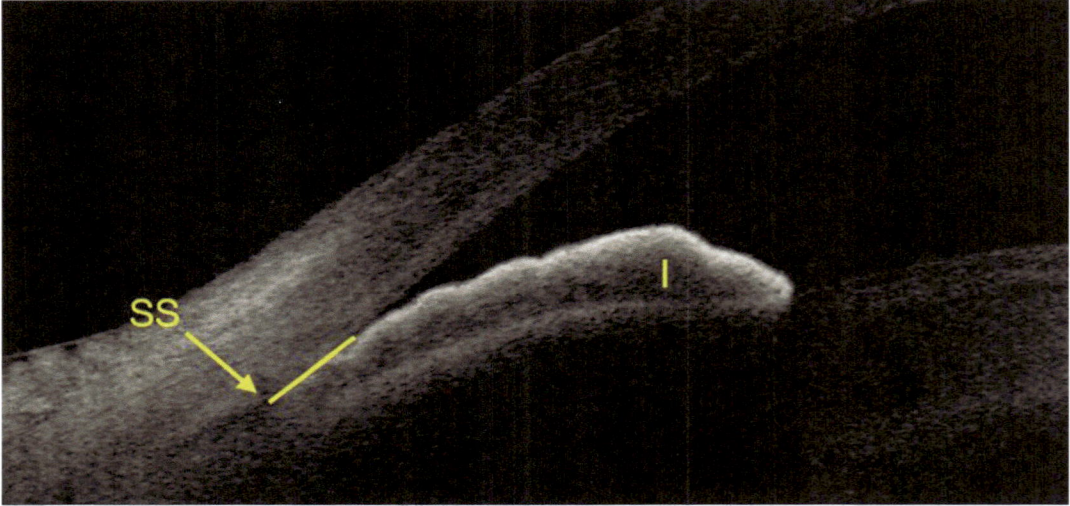

Fig. 1.5 Image taken with the Tomey CASIA SS-1000 demonstrating angle closure. Scleral spur (SS, yellow arrow), iris (I), and segment of iridotrabecular contact (yellow line) are marked

Anatomically, the trabecular meshwork is bounded anteriorly by Schwalbe's line and posteriorly by the scleral spur. As angle closure tends to start posteriorly near the iris root and progress anteriorly, the key anatomical structure to identify in the interpretation of AS-OCT images is the scleral spur. The scleral spur lies at the junction of the trabecular meshwork and ciliary body. On AS-OCT images, the scleral spur is defined as the inward protrusion of the sclera where a change in curvature of the corneoscleral junction is observed (Fig. 1.6) [28]. One AS-OCT study found the average width of the trabecular meshwork ranges between 712 and 889 μm in width depending on the portion of the angle being imaged [29]. Therefore, AS-OCT parameters developed to measure angle width typically focus on a region 250 to 1000 μm anterior to the scleral spur.

Schwalbe's line has been proposed as an alternative to the scleral spur as a reference landmark for measuring AS-OCT parameters [30, 31]. Schwalbe's line is more visible and reliably identified on spectral-domain AS-OCT imaging (Fig. 1.7) [7]. In addition, parameters such as

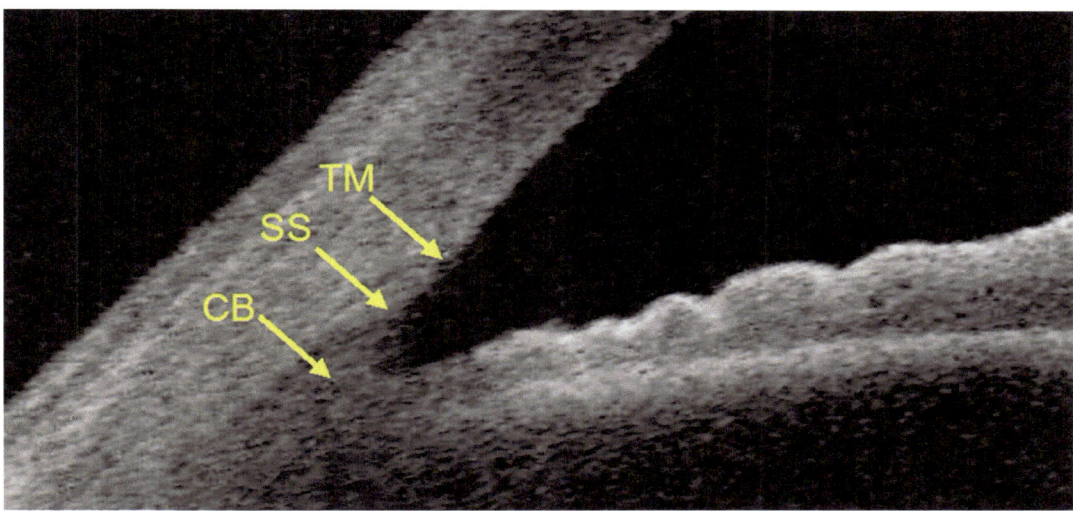

Fig. 1.6 Image taken with the Tomey CASIA SS-1000 demonstrating the scleral spur (SS) located at the junction of the trabecular meshwork (TM) and ciliary body (CB)

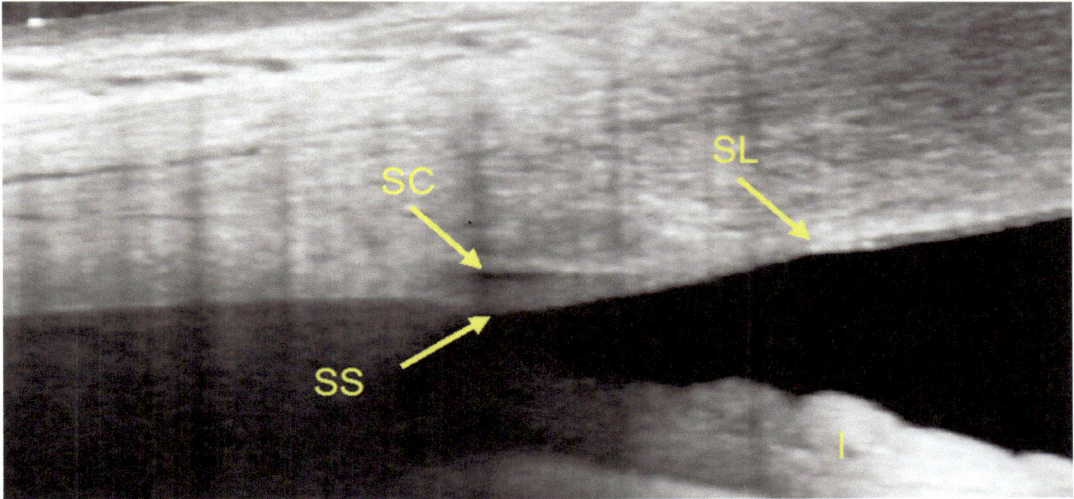

Fig. 1.7 Image taken with the Heidelberg Spectralis with anterior segment module. The iris (I), Schwalbe's line (SL, yellow arrow), Scleral spur (SS, yellow arrow) and Schlemm's canal (SC, yellow arrow) are marked

AOD measured at the location of Schwalbe's line are highly correlated with gonioscopic angle closure [31, 32]. However, the scleral spur currently remains the reference landmark in the majority of AS-OCT studies, both for historical reasons and given the close proximity of its anatomical location to the trabecular meshwork.

As mentioned previously, the primary objective of the examiner is to identify the scleral spur and assess if there is contact between the iris and corneoscleral junction anterior to this point. It is important to note that angle closure defined in this manner based on AS-OCT images is not equivalent to gonioscopic angle closure, which is typically defined as the inability to visualize pigmented trabecular meshwork on gonioscopy. In fact, there is only weak agreement between AS-OCT and gonioscopy in the detection and assessment of angle closure [4, 33]. Therefore, the two assessment methods should not be used interchangeably.

Rather, AS-OCT imaging provides complementary information to gonioscopy in patients in whom appositional angle closure is suspected.

Detection of the scleral spur is more difficult in eyes with angle closure due to crowding of the iridocorneal angle by iris tissue and attenuation of OCT signal (Fig. 1.8). However, with training and experience, it can be detected at a high rate on modern AS-OCT devices as long as the eyelid is adequately retracted during the time of imaging [7]. Disparities in the detection of angle closure between AS-OCT and gonioscopy likely arise from influences of ocular structures, such as the iris and lens, to visualization of angle structures on gonioscopy (Fig. 1.9). For example, Fig. 1.9 illustrates a case in which angle closure was diagnosed on gonioscopy but was not corroborated by AS-OCT imaging. In this case, there is significant anterior positioning of the lens and bowing of the iris, both of which affect the examiner's ability to visualize the pigmented trabecular meshwork.

AS-OCT images can also be interpreted quantitatively, although this requires specialized software not available on all AS-OCT devices. Some AS-OCT devices, such as the Tomey CASIA, have robust built-in software for measuring the width of the angle, extent of iridotrabecular contact (ITC) anterior to the scleral spur, and dimensions of the anterior chamber and its structures (Fig. 1.10) [34]. Other devices, such as the Heidelberg Spectralis, have more limited measurement tools, although these are not FDA approved for patient care or activated on most devices. On the Tomey CASIA, ocular structures such as the cornea, lens, or iris must first be delineated, either automatically by the software or manually by the user. Then, the scleral spur must be marked before measurements of AS-OCT parameters can be computed. This process tends to be time-consuming, which has limited the clinical utility of quantitative AS-OCT measurements. In addition, there is currently no commercially available software for computing AS-OCT

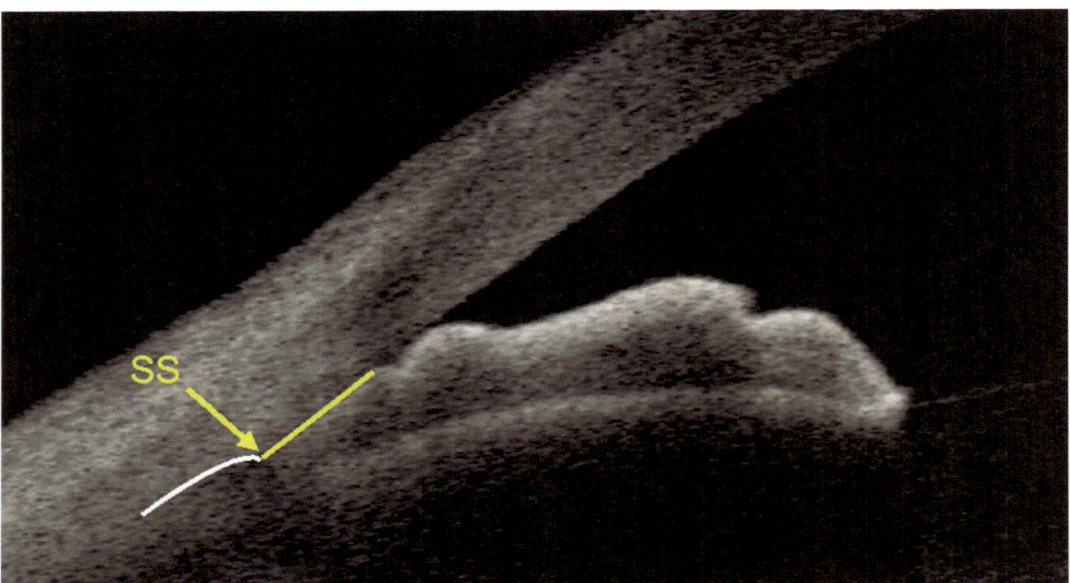

Fig. 1.8 Image taken with the Tomey CASIA SS-1000 demonstrating difficulty of identifying the scleral spur in an eye with angle closure. The scleral spur (SS, yellow arrow), segment of iridotrabecular contact (yellow line), and faint outline of the junction between the sclera and ciliary body (white line) are marked

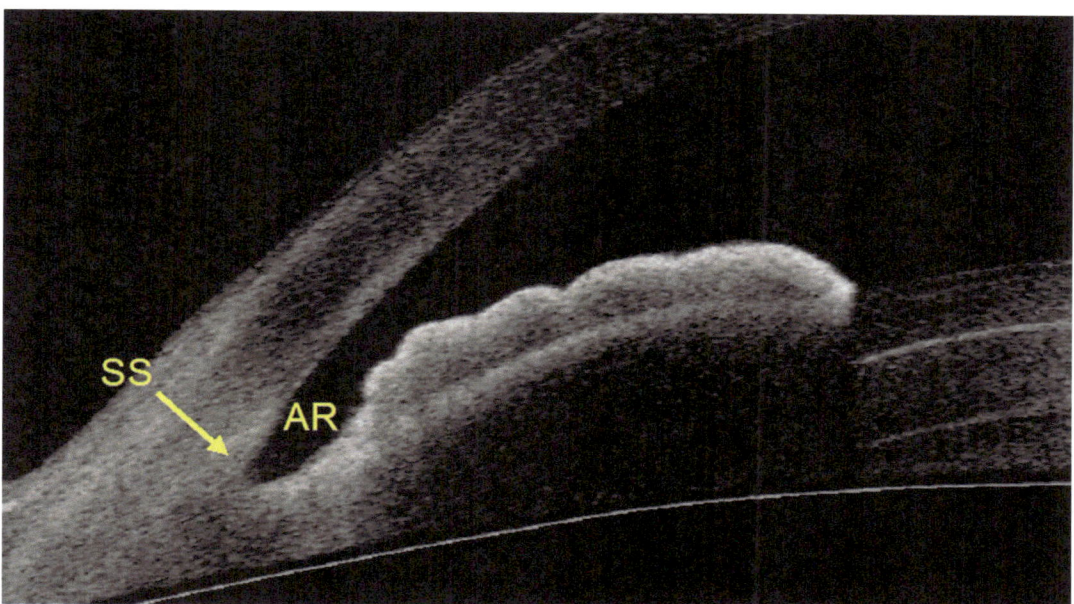

Fig. 1.9 Image taken with the Tomey CASIA SS-1000 demonstrating a lack of iridotrabecular contact in the angle recess (AR) anterior to the scleral spur (SS, yellow arrow) in angle quadrant diagnosed with gonioscopic angle closure

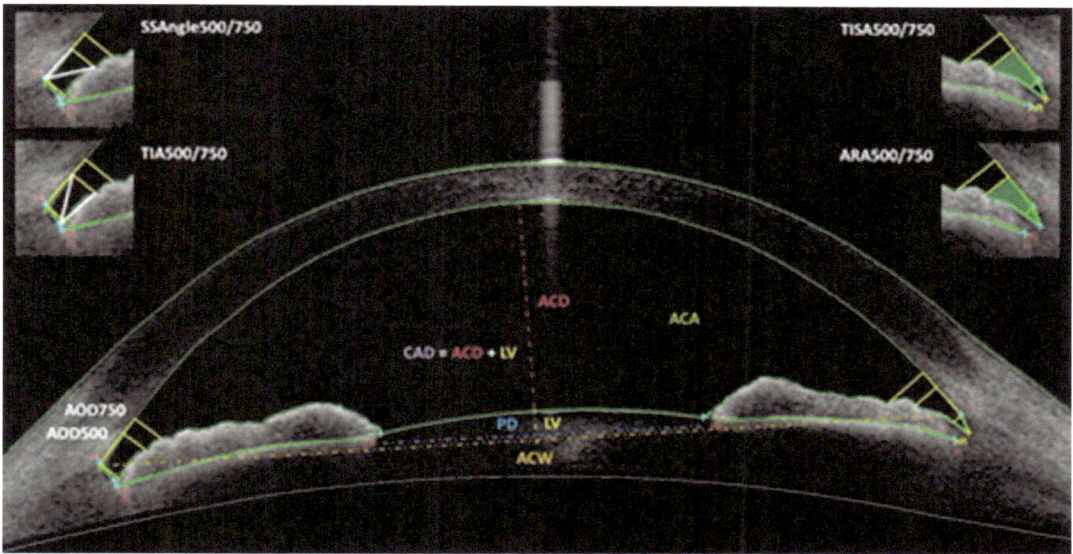

Fig. 1.10 Anterior segment parameters measured by Tomey CASIA SS-1000 using manufacturer-provided software. AOD: angle opening distance. ARA: angle recess area. TIA: trabecular iris angle. TISA: trabecular iris space area. SSAngle: scleral spur angle. ACD: anterior chamber depth. LV: lens vault. CAD: corneal arcuate distance. ACW: anterior chamber width. PD: pupillary diameter. ACA: anterior chamber area. 500 and 750 denote distance from scleral spur in µm

measurements from a variety of AS-OCT devices. AS-OCT studies of the iridocorneal angle reveal significant anatomical variation [10]. While most of this anatomical variation is missed by a single cross-sectional image along the horizontal temporal-nasal meridian, it is captured by as few as four OCT images on average [9, 10]. Therefore, a multi-image analysis approach is recommended for quantitative studies of angle width.

AS-OCT parameters have been devised to describe the dimensions of the iridocorneal angle (Fig. 1.10). The most commonly measured angle parameters include angle opening distance (AOD), angle recess area (ARA), trabecular iris space area (TISA), trabecular iris angle (TIA), and scleral spur angle (SSA) measured at 500 and 750 μm from the scleral spur. AOD is calculated as the perpendicular distance measured from the trabecular meshwork at 500 or 750 μm anterior to the scleral spur to the anterior iris surface. ARA is the area of the angle recess bounded anteriorly by the AOD. TISA is an area bound anteriorly by AOD, posteriorly by a line drawn from the scleral spur perpendicular to the plane of the inner scleral wall to the opposing iris, superiorly by the inner corneoscleral wall, and inferiorly by the iris surface. TIA and SSA are defined as an angle measured with the apex in the iris recess or at the scleral spur, respectively, and the arms of the angle passing through a point on the trabecular meshwork 500 or 750 μm from the scleral spur and the point on the iris perpendicularly. Parameters measuring angle width have a direct relationship with gonioscopy grades or PACD status, although this relationship differs between eyes with open angles and angle closure [35, 36]. Other AS-OCT parameters that describe the dimensions of the anterior chamber and its structures, such as lens vault (LV) and anterior chamber area (ACA), have been identified as biometric risk factors for PACD. These will be discussed in the next section *Biometric Risk Factors for Angle Closure*.

When performing AS-OCT imaging, there are two important factors to take into account: standardization of lighting conditions and retraction of the eyelid. Pupil diameter, a strong determinant of angle width, is affected by environmental lighting conditions due to the pupillary light reflex. Small changes in pupil size can have large effects on angle width measured by AS-OCT [37]. Therefore, it is important to standardize lighting conditions, if not pupil size, during AS-OCT imaging. In addition, inadequate retraction of the eyelid can lead to attenuation of signal, which makes it difficult or impossible to identify the anatomical structures of the iridocorneal angle (Fig. 1.11).

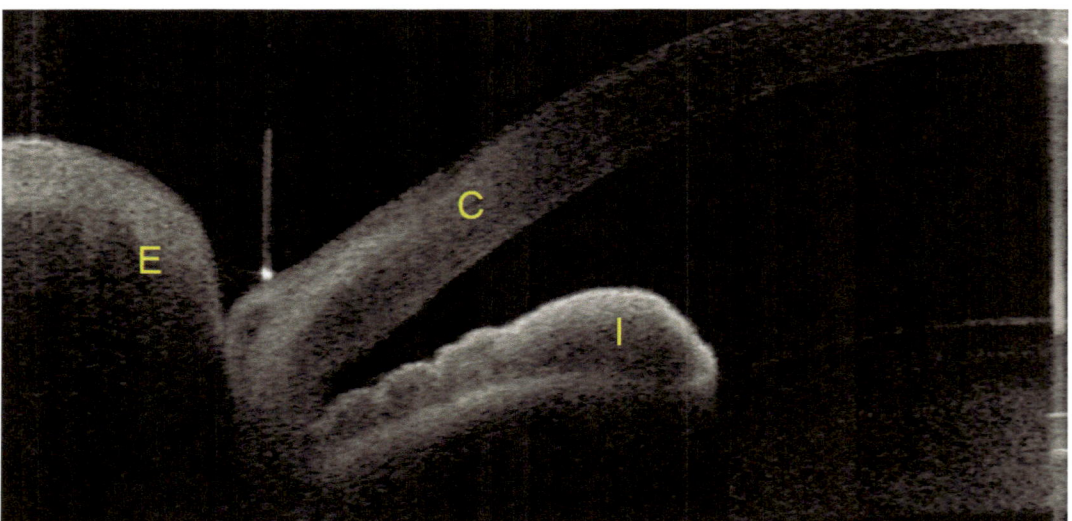

Fig. 1.11 Image taken with the Tomey CASIA SS-1000 demonstrating effect of inadequate eyelid retraction during time of imaging. Eyelid (E), cornea (C), and iris (I) are marked. The scleral spur cannot be reliably identified in this image

Biometric Risk Factors for Angle Closure

Angle closure refers to mechanical obstruction of the trabecular meshwork by the peripheral iris. Angle closure leads to impaired aqueous outflow and elevations in IOP, a strong risk factor for glaucomatous optic neuropathy. Primary angle closure disease (PACD) broadly refers to individuals at risk for this process and is typically divided based on the following gonioscopic classification system [38].

- Primary angle closure suspect (PACS), defined as having gonioscopic angle closure in three or more quadrants without evidence of trabecular meshwork dysfunction or glaucomatous optic neuropathy
- Primary angle closure (PAC), defined as PACS with peripheral anterior synechiae (PAS), excessive pigment deposition on the trabecular meshwork, or elevated IOP > 21 mmHg
- Primary angle closure glaucoma (PACG), defined as PAC with glaucomatous optic neuropathy

Angle parameters that directly measure angle width are intuitive risk factors for gonioscopic angle closure and PACD. However, studies have also identified non-angle parameters that are associated with angle closure. These biometric risk factors can be divided into two categories: static, which comprise measurements derived from individual AS-OCT images, and dynamic, which are measurements computed by comparing measurements from two AS-OCT images, typically obtained under different environmental conditions. Static risk factors include lens vault, anterior chamber area and volume, and iris thickness, area, and curvature [39–44]. Dynamic risk factors include changes in iris area in response to changes in pupil diameter [42–44].

Static Risk Factors

The strongest and most consistently reported static risk factor for gonioscopic angle closure is lens vault (LV), defined as the perpendicular distance separating the anterior pole of the lens from an imaginary horizontal line joining the two scleral spurs [39–42]. Larger values of lens vault are suggestive of increased crowding of the anterior chamber and iridocorneal angle by a thicker or more anterior lens (Fig. 1.12). One study examining angle closure in Chinese subjects reported a

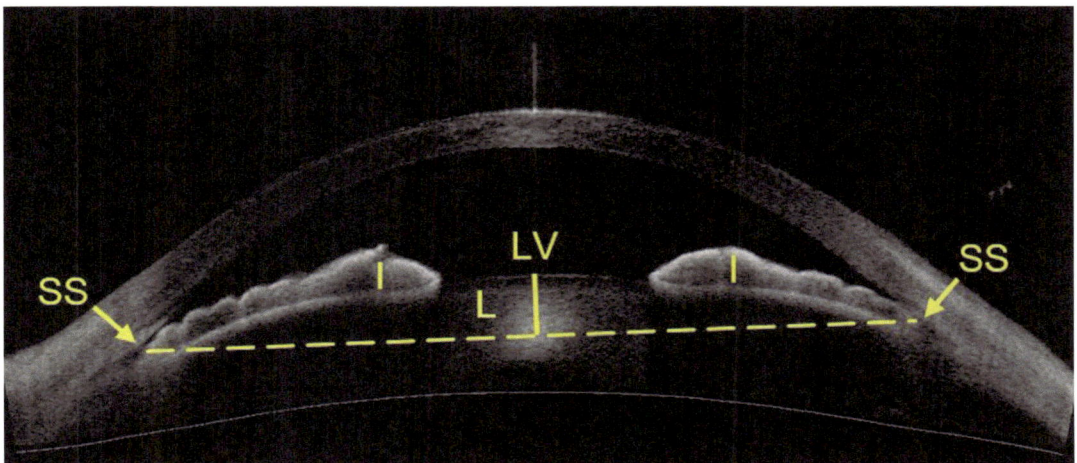

Fig. 1.12 Image taken with the Tomey CASIA SS-1000 demonstrating eye with increased lens vault and angle closure. The iris appears anteriorly bowed and draped over the lens. Scleral spurs (SS), scleral spur plane (dashed yellow line), iris (I), lens (L), and lens vault (LV, yellow line) are marked

significant correlation between gonioscopic angle closure and lens vault [39]. Specifically, eyes in the highest quartile of lens vault measurements were at 48 times higher risk of angle closure compared to subjects in the lowest quartile. This association was independent of known non-biometric risk factors, such as age and gender, as well as other biometric risk factors, such as anterior chamber depth, lens thickness, and relative lens position. These findings were corroborated by a study of Japanese subjects, which reported an odds ratio of 24.2 for angle closure when comparing the lowest and highest quartiles of lens vault measurements [40].

A number of iris-related AS-OCT parameters have also been described as biometric risk factors for angle closure [41–43]. Iris thickness (IT), defined as the largest perpendicular distance along the iris connecting the anterior and posterior iris borders, was found to have an odds ratio of 2.2–2.7 for angle closure when compared with normal eyes. Iris curvature (IC), defined as the perpendicular distance between the iris pigment epithelium and an imaginary line connecting the most peripheral and most central points of iris pigment epithelium, at the point of greatest convexity, and iris area (IA), defined as the cross-sectional area of the full length of the iris, were found to have odds ratios of 0.4–2.5 and 1.1–2.7, respectively.

AS-OCT measurements describing the anterior chamber have also been studied as biometric predictors for angle closure disease. Smaller anterior chamber area (ACA), defined as the cross-sectional area bounded by the corneal endothelium, anterior surface of iris, and anterior surface of lens within the pupil and smaller anterior chamber volume (ACV), calculated by rotating the anterior chamber area 360 degrees around a vertical axis drawn through the midpoint of the anterior chamber, were found to have odds ratios of 53.2 and 40.2, respectively [44]. This translates into 89.9% sensitivity and 85.5% specificity if anterior chamber area measured by AS-OCT is used as a screening parameter for PACD.

Multiparameter models aggregate information provided by multiple biometric risk factors to make predictions on the status of the iridocorneal angle.

A six-parameter model based on LV, IA, IT, ACA, ACV, and anterior chamber width (ACW) can generate a probability estimate for gonioscopic angle closure with an area under the receiver operating characteristic curve (AUC) value of 0.94 [49]. A separate longitudinal study that examined the ability of AS-OCT parameters to predicted gonioscopic angle closure reported a model consisting of AOD750 and LV explained 38% of variance in gonioscopic angle closure occurring at 4 years [50]. These results suggest there is a complementary benefit to analyzing multiple biometric risk factors, although there is redundancy in the predictive information they provide.

Dynamic Risk Factors

Dynamic risk factors for angle closure primarily currently focus on changes in the iris associated with pupillary dilation. Studies have shown behaviors of the iris in the transition between light and dark environments differ significantly between open angle and angle closure eyes. Early studies used AS-OCT to quantify and compare the changes in iris area and iris volume associated with pupillary dilation in angle closure versus open angle subjects [45–48]. The results revealed a smaller decrease of iris area and volume with dilation in angle closure eyes compared to open angle eyes.

A more recent study found larger, more peripherally distributed irises increase the risk of post-dilation angle closure [41]. PACS and PACG subjects demonstrated less loss of iris area per millimeter of pupillary distance (PD) increase after physiologic dilation when compared with normal subjects. Regression analysis confirmed that less iris area loss per millimeter PD increase was a significant risk factor for an occludable angle, defined as non-visibility of posterior trabecular meshwork for at least 180 degrees. Furthermore, the change in centroid-to-centroid distance (CCD), defined as the distance between the centers of the nasal and temporal iris masses, per millimeter of PD increase was significantly greater in PACS and PACG subjects compared with normal subjects.

Treatments for Angle Closure and Glaucoma

Glaucoma treatments include lasers procedures and incisional surgeries. More recently, incisional surgery has been subdivided into minimally invasive glaucoma surgery (MIGS) and traditional invasive surgery (e.g., trabeculectomy and glaucoma tube shunts). These interventions are administered in conjunction with medical therapies to control IOP in patients with progressive glaucomatous damage. One role proposed for AS-OCT has been for guiding and evaluating the outcomes of these glaucoma treatments.

Laser peripheral iridotomy (LPI) is typically the first-line intervention in the treatment of angle closure to widen the iridocorneal angle and alleviate angle closure. This procedure utilizes an Nd:YAG laser to create a full-thickness hole in the iris that provides aqueous with an alternative outflow pathway from the posterior chamber to the anterior chamber. LPI significantly increases angle width in angle closure eyes as measured by AS-OCT parameters such as AOD500, TISA500, and ARA500 [51–53]. However, the use of LPI varies widely in early stage PACD as there is no widely held consensus on when it should be performed in the absence of PAS, elevated IOP, or glaucomatous optic neuropathy.

Progressive enlargement of the crystalline lens contributes to pupillary block, the primary mechanism underlying angle closure and PACD. Cataract extraction can widen the angle and lower IOP [54–56]. In angle closure eyes, postsurgical decreases in IOP are primarily due to improved access to the conventional outflow pathway by the aqueous humor. However, AS-OCT studies have also shown that dilations of Schlemm's canal are observable after phacoemulsification surgery, which may explain its IOP-lowering effect even in eyes with open angles [27, 55]. Phacoemulsification combined with goniosynechialysis is often considered as the primary surgical intervention to alleviate angle closure and lower IOP in patients with PACG [57]. The addition of goniosynechialysis provides greater reduction of iridotrabecular contact than phacoemulsification alone, a beneficial effect that can be quantified by AS-OCT. [28]

The well-established gold standard in glaucoma surgery is trabeculectomy, which creates a corneoscleral opening under a partial-thickness scleral flap. This opening serves as an alternate pathway for aqueous outflow from the anterior chamber to the sub-Tenon's and sub-conjunctival spaces, leading to the formation of a bleb. AS-OCT provides detailed visualization of the trabeculectomy bleb (Fig. 1.13), and several stud-

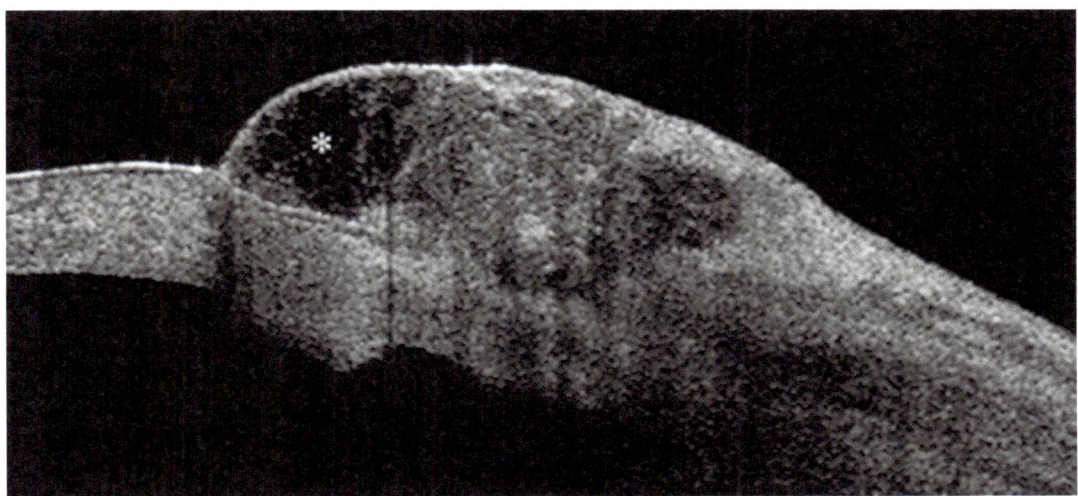

Fig. 1.13 Image taken with the Zeiss Visante demonstrating functioning filtering bleb after MMC-augmented trabeculectomy. The multilobed cystic bleb shows a pat- ent and low reflective fluid-filled inner cavity (asterisk) (Reprinted from Mastropasqua et al., 2014 under a Creative Commons Attribution license [64])

ies have reported an association of bleb morphology with level of IOP control [58–64]. Features of bleb morphology associated with successful IOP lowering include a multilayered appearance and low reflectivity of the bleb wall, presence of episcleral fluid, as well as lower internal reflectivity of the fluid-filled cavity [62, 63]. AS-OCT can also be used to quantify dynamic changes in bleb morphology following laser suture lysis, which can be predictive of long-term surgical outcome [65, 66].

A number of minimally invasive glaucoma surgeries (MIGS) have been introduced over the past decade for the surgical management of glaucoma patients. MIGS devices restore, enhance, or provide an alternative to the eye's natural aqueous outflow pathways by shunting aqueous from the anterior chamber into Schlemm's canal, suprachoroidal space, or sub-Tenon's and subconjunctival spaces. AS-OCT imaging provides a noninvasive method to evaluate short- and long-term postsurgical placement and effect of MIGS in these anatomical structures and spaces [25, 67–70].

Future Directions of Research

AS-OCT technology has rapidly evolved over the past decade. However, the clinical adoption of AS-OCT imaging for the management of PACD has been slow. One reason is there are no automated methods to facilitate the quantitative interpretation of AS-OCT images. Another reason is that clinical and functional significance of angle closure detected by AS-OCT imaging is not as well understood as the significance of angle closure detected by gonioscopy.

The primary advantage of AS-OCT over gonioscopy is it provides quantitative measurements in addition to qualitative assessments of angle width. Automated algorithms support the quantitative analyses of posterior segment structures, such as the retina and optic nerve head. Longitudinal measurements of retinal and nerve fiber layer thickness have modernized the management of posterior segment diseases, allowing clinicians to detect disease progression and response to treatment. In theory, AS-OCT could

support similar longitudinal studies of anterior segment diseases. However, quantitative analysis of AS-OCT images is at best semiautomated and requires manual identification of the scleral spur in each image [71]. Experimental automated methods that extract measurements from AS-OCT images by matching them to hand-marked exemplar datasets demonstrated only satisfactory performance [72]. AS-OCT measurements could be used to detect the presence or progression of anterior segment diseases, including PACD [49, 73]. However, clinical adoption of quantitative AS-OCT imaging will likely remain limited until well-performing automated methods have been integrated into mainstream commercial AS-OCT devices.

The current AS-OCT definition of angle closure is based on static structural findings lacking long-term clinical and functional significance. AS-OCT imaging provides three-dimensional information about the structural configuration of the iridocorneal angle, which reflects the amount of access aqueous humor has to the conventional outflow pathway. However, studies exploring this structure-function relationship are limited. One recent study explored the relationship between average angle width measured by AS-OCT and IOP and established threshold values below which angle width and IOP are strongly correlated [74]. However, the degree and extent of iridotrabecular contact required before aqueous outflow and IOP are affected is unknown. Longitudinal studies of angle closure detected on AS-OCT are similarly limited. One study found that in eyes with open angles on baseline examination, iridotrabecular contact detected on AS-OCT was predictive of gonioscopic angle closure after 4 years [75]. Therefore, future research must focus on developing functionally significant definitions of angle closure that are validated through longitudinal clinical studies.

Conclusion

AS-OCT is a noninvasive in vivo imaging method that has gained popularity among clinicians and researchers over the past decade. AS-OCT imaging facilitates qualitative and quantitative studies of the anterior segment and has applications for characterizing anatomical structures, diagnosing and staging disease, and assessing treatment efficacy. However, its adoption in routine clinical care significantly lags behind OCT studies of the posterior segment. Therefore, further work is needed to demonstrate and validate the benefit of novel OCT-based methods compared to current clinical standards of care in the management of anterior segment diseases.

Compliance with Ethical Requirements Benjamin Y. Xu, Jing Shan, Charles DeBoer, and Tin Aung declare that they have no conflicts of interest. No human or animal studies were carried out by the authors for this article.

References

1. Izatt JA, Hee MR, Swanson EA, et al. Micrometer-scale resolution imaging of the anterior eye in vivo with optical coherence tomography. Arch Ophthalmol. 1994;112(12):1584–9.
2. Asrani S, Sarunic M, Santiago C, Izatt J. Detailed visualization of the anterior segment using Fourier-domain optical coherence tomography. Arch Ophthalmol. 2008;126(6):765–71.
3. Liu S, Yu M, Ye C, Lam DSC, Leung CKS. Anterior chamber angle imaging with swept-source optical coherence tomography: An investigation on variability of angle measurement. Investig Ophthalmol Vis Sci. 2011;52(12):8598–603.
4. Sakata LM, Lavanya R, Friedman DS, et al. Comparison of Gonioscopy and anterior segment ocular coherence tomography in detecting angle closure in different quadrants of the anterior chamber angle. Ophthalmology. 2008;115(5):769–74.
5. Sharma R, Sharma A, Arora T, et al. Application of anterior segment optical coherence tomography in glaucoma. Surv Ophthalmol. 2014;59(3):311–27.
6. Maram J, Pan X, Sadda S, Francis B, Marion K, Chopra V. Reproducibility of angle metrics using the time-domain anterior segment optical coherence tomography: intra-observer and inter-observer variability. Curr Eye Res. 2015;40(5):496–500.
7. McKee H, Ye C, Yu M, Liu S, Lam DSC, Leung CKS. Anterior chamber angle imaging with swept-source optical coherence tomography: detecting the scleral spur, Schwalbe's line, and Schlemm's canal. J Glaucoma. 2013;22(6):468–72.
8. Pan X, Marion K, Maram J, et al. Reproducibility of anterior segment angle metrics measurements derived from cirrus spectral domain optical coherence tomography. J Glaucoma. 2015;24(5):e47–51.
9. Blieden LS, Chuang AZ, Baker LA, et al. Optimal number of angle images for calculating anterior angle volume and iris volume measurements. Investig Ophthalmol Vis Sci. 2015;56(5):2842–7.
10. Xu BY, Israelsen P, Pan BX, Wang D, Jiang X, Varma R. Benefit of measuring anterior segment structures using an increased number of optical coherence tomography images: the Chinese American Eye Study. Investig Ophthalmol Vis Sci. 2016;57(14):6313–9.
11. Aptel F, Chiquet C, Gimbert A, et al. Anterior segment biometry using spectral-domain optical coherence tomography. J Refract Surg. 2014;30(5):354–60.
12. Marion KM, Maram J, Pan X, et al. Reproducibility and agreement between 2 spectral domain optical coherence tomography devices for anterior chamber angle measurements. J Glaucoma. 2015;24(9):642–6.
13. Cumba RJ, Radhakrishnan S, Bell NP, et al. Reproducibility of scleral spur identification and angle measurements using fourier domain anterior segment optical coherence tomography. J Ophthalmol. 2012;2012:1–14.
14. Xu BY, Mai DD, Penteado RC, Saunders L, Weinreb RN. Reproducibility and agreement of anterior segment parameter measurements obtained using the CASIA2 and Spectralis OCT2 optical coherence tomography devices. J Glaucoma. 2017;26(11):974–9.
15. Akil H, Dastiridou A, Marion K, Francis B, Chopra V. Repeatability, reproducibility, agreement characteristics of 2 SD-OCT devices for anterior chamber angle measurements. Can J Ophthalmol. 2017;52(2):166–70.
16. Foster PJ, Aung T, Nolan WP, et al. Defining "occludable" angles in population surveys: drainage angle width, peripheral anterior synechiae, and glaucomatous optic neuropathy in east Asian people. Br J Ophthalmol. 2004;88(4):486–90.
17. Rigi M, Bell NP, Lee DA, et al. Agreement between Gonioscopic examination and swept source Fourier domain anterior segment optical coherence tomography imaging. J Ophthalmol. 2016;2016:1727039.
18. Tello C, Liebmann J, Potash SD, Cohen H, Ritch R. Measurement of ultrasound biomicroscopy images: intraobserver and interobserver reliability. Invest Ophthalmol Vis Sci. 1994;35(9):3549–52.
19. Spaeth GL, Azuara-Blanco A, Araujo SV, Augsburger JJ. Intraobserver and interobserver agreement in evaluating the anterior chamber angle configuration by ultrasound biomicroscopy. J Glaucoma. 1997;6(1):13–7.
20. Huang AS, Belghith A, Dastiridou A, Chopra V, Zangwill LM, Weinreb RN. Automated circumferential construction of first-order aqueous humor outflow pathways using spectral-domain optical coherence tomography. J Biomed Opt. 2017;22(6):66010.
21. Li P, An L, Reif R, Shen TT, Johnstone M, Wang RK. In vivo microstructural and microvascular imaging of the human corneo-scleral limbus using optical coherence tomography. Biomed Opt Express. 2011;2(11):3109–18.

22. Uji A, Muraoka Y, Yoshimura N. In vivo identification of the Posttrabecular aqueous outflow pathway using swept-source optical coherence tomography. Investig Opthalmol Vis Sci. 2016;57(10):4162.

23. Huang AS, Camp A, Xu BY, Penteado RC, Weinreb RN. Aqueous angiography: aqueous humor outflow imaging in live human subjects. Ophthalmology. 2017;124(8):1249–51.

24. Gazzard G, Friedman DS, Devereux J, Sean S. Primary acute angle closure glaucoma associated with suprachoroidal fluid in three Chinese patients. Eye. 2001;15(3):358–60.

25. Saheb H, Ianchulev T, Ahmed IK. Optical coherence tomography of the suprachoroid after CyPass Micro-Stent implantation for the treatment of open-angle glaucoma. Br J Ophthalmol. 2014;98(1):19–23.

26. Vieira L, Noronha M, Lemos V, Reina M, Gomes T. Anterior segment optical coherence tomography imaging of filtering blebs after deep Sclerectomy with Esnoper-clip implant: one-year follow-up. J Curr Glaucoma Pract. 2014;8(3):91–5.

27. Zhao Z, Zhu X, He W, Jiang C, Lu Y. Schlemm's canal expansion after uncomplicated phacoemulsification surgery: an optical coherence tomography study. Investig Ophthalmol Vis Sci. 2016;57(15):6507–12.

28. Ho SW, Baskaran M, Zheng C, et al. Swept source optical coherence tomography measurement of the iris-trabecular contact (ITC) index: a new parameter for angle closure. Graefes Arch Clin Exp Ophthalmol. 2013;251(4):1205–11.

29. Tun TA, Baskaran M, Zheng C, et al. Assessment of trabecular meshwork width using swept source optical coherence tomography. Graefes Arch Clin Exp Ophthalmol. 2013;251(6):1587–92.

30. Cheung CY, Zheng C, Ho C-L, et al. Novel anterior-chamber angle measurements by high-definition optical coherence tomography using the Schwalbe line as the landmark. Br J Ophthalmol. 2011;95(7):955–9.

31. Qin B, Francis BA, Li Y, et al. Anterior chamber angle measurements using Schwalbe's line with high-resolution Fourier-domain optical coherence tomography. J Glaucoma. 2013;22(9):684–8.

32. Cheung CY, Zheng C, Ho CL, et al. Novel anterior-chamber angle measurements by high-definition optical coherence tomography using the Schwalbe line as the landmark. Br J Ophthalmol. 2011;95(7):955–9.

33. Xu BY, Pardeshi AA, Burkemper B, et al. Quantitative evaluation of Gonioscopic and EyeCam assessments of angle dimensions using anterior segment optical coherence tomography. Transl Vis Sci Technol. 2018;7(6):33.

34. Baskaran M, Ho S-W, Tun TA, et al. Assessment of circumferential angle-closure by the iris-trabecular contact index with swept-source optical coherence tomography. Ophthalmology. 2013;120(11):2226–31.

35. Narayanaswamy A, Sakata LM, He MG, et al. Diagnostic performance of anterior chamber angle measurements for detecting eyes with narrow angles: an anterior segment OCT study. Arch Ophthalmol. 2010;128(10):1321–7.

36. Xu BY, Pardeshi AA, Burkemper B, et al. Quantitative evaluation of Gonioscopic and EyeCam assessments of angle dimensions using anterior segment optical coherence tomography. Transl Vis Sci Technol. 2018;7(6):33.

37. Leung CKS, Cheung CYL, Li H, et al. Dynamic analysis of dark-light changes of the anterior chamber angle with anterior segment OCT. Investig Ophthalmol Vis Sci. 2007;48(9):4116–22.

38. Foster PJ, Buhrmann R, Quigley HA, Johnson GJ. The definition and classification of glaucoma in prevalence surveys. Br J Ophthalmol. 2002;86(2):238–42.

39. Nongpiur ME, He M, Amerasinghe N, et al. Lens vault, thickness, and position in Chinese subjects with angle closure. Ophthalmology. 2011;118(3):474–9.

40. Ozaki M, Nongpiur ME, Aung T, He M, Mizoguchi T. Increased lens vault as a risk factor for angle closure: confirmation in a Japanese population. Graefes Arch Clin Exp Ophthalmol. 2012;250(12):1863–8.

41. Zhang Y, Li SZ, Li L, He MG, Thomas R, Wang NL. Dynamic iris changes as a risk factor in primary angle closure disease. Investig Ophthalmol Vis Sci. 2016;57(1):218–26.

42. Wang B, Sakata LM, Friedman DS, et al. Quantitative Iris parameters and association with narrow angles. Ophthalmology. 2010;117(1):11–7.

43. Wang BS, Narayanaswamy A, Amerasinghe N, et al. Increased iris thickness and association with primary angle closure glaucoma. Br J Ophthalmol. 2011;95(1):46–50.

44. Wu RY, Nongpiur ME, He MG, et al. Association of narrow angles with anterior chamber area and volume measured with anterior-segment optical coherence tomography. Arch Ophthalmol. 2011;129(5):569–74.

45. Aptel F, Chiquet C, Beccat S, Denis P. Biometric evaluation of anterior chamber changes after physiologic pupil dilation using Pentacam and anterior segment optical coherence tomography. Investig Ophthalmol Vis Sci. 2012;53(7):4005–10.

46. Aptel F, Denis P. Optical coherence tomography quantitative analysis of Iris volume changes after pharmacologic Mydriasis. Ophthalmology. 2010;117(1):3–10.

47. Quigley HA, Silver DM, Friedman DS, et al. Iris cross-sectional area decreases with pupil dilation and its dynamic behavior is a risk factor in angle closure. J Glaucoma. 2009;18(3):173–9.

48. Seager FE, Jefferys JL, Quigley HA. Comparison of dynamic changes in anterior ocular structures examined with anterior segment optical coherence tomography in a cohort of various origins. Investig Ophthalmol Vis Sci. 2014;55(3):1672–83.

49. Nongpiur ME, Haaland BA, Perera SA, et al. Development of a score and probability estimate for detecting angle closure based on anterior segment optical coherence tomography. Am J Ophthalmol. 2014;157(1):32–38.e1.

50. Nongpiur ME, Aboobakar IF, Baskaran M, et al. Association of baseline anterior segment parameters

with the development of incident Gonioscopic angle closure. JAMA Ophthalmol. 2017;135(3):252–8.

51. Ramakrishnan R, Mitra A, Abdul Kader M, Das S. To study the efficacy of laser peripheral iridoplasty in the treatment of eyes with primary angle closure and plateau iris syndrome, unresponsive to laser peripheral iridotomy, using anterior-segment OCT as a tool. J Glaucoma. 2016;25(5):440–6.

52. Lee KS, Sung KR, Kang SY, Cho JW, Kim DY, Kook MS. Residual anterior chamber angle closure in narrow-angle eyes following laser peripheral iridotomy: anterior segment optical coherence tomography quantitative study. Jpn J Ophthalmol. 2011;55(3):213–9.

53. Radhakrishnan S, Chen PP, Junk AK, Nouri-Mahdavi K, Chen TC. Laser peripheral Iridotomy in primary angle closure: a report by the American Academy of Ophthalmology. Ophthalmology. 2018;125(7):1110–20.

54. Harasymowycz PJ, Papamatheakis DG, Ahmed I, et al. Phacoemulsification and goniosynechialysis in the management of unresponsive primary angle closure. J Glaucoma. 2005;14(3):186–9.

55. Mansberger SL, Gordon MO, Jampel H, et al. Reduction in intraocular pressure after cataract extraction: the ocular hypertension treatment study. Ophthalmology. 2012;119(9):1826–31.

56. Zhang ZM, Niu Q, Nie Y, Zhang J. Reduction of intraocular pressure and improvement of vision after cataract surgeries in angle closure glaucoma with concomitant cataract patients. Int J Clin Exp Med. 2015;8(9):16557–63.

57. Tham CCY, Kwong YYY, Baig N, Leung DYL, Li FCH, Lam DSC. Phacoemulsification versus trabeculectomy in medically uncontrolled chronic angle-closure glaucoma without cataract. Ophthalmology. 2013;120(1):62–7.

58. Singh M, Chew PTK, Friedman DS, et al. Imaging of trabeculectomy blebs using anterior segment optical coherence tomography. Ophthalmology. 2007;114(1):47–53.

59. Savini G, Zanini M, Barboni P. Filtering blebs imaging by optical coherence tomography. Clin Exp Ophthalmol. 2005;33(5):483–9.

60. Inoue T, Matsumura R, Kuroda U, Nakashima KI, Kawaji T, Tanihara H. Precise identification of filtration openings on the scleral flap by three-dimensional anterior segment optical coherence tomography. Investig Ophthalmol Vis Sci. 2012;53(13):8288–94.

61. Nakano N, Hangai M, Nakanishi H, et al. Early trabeculectomy bleb walls on anterior-segment optical coherence tomography. Graefes Arch Clin Exp Ophthalmol. 2010;248(8):1173–82.

62. Pfenninger L, Schneider F, Funk J. Internal reflectivity of filtering blebs versus intraocular pressure in patients with recent trabeculectomy. Investig Ophthalmol Vis Sci. 2011;52(5):2450–5.

63. Tominaga A, Miki A, Yamazaki Y, Matsushita K, Otori Y. The assessment of the filtering bleb function with anterior segment optical coherence tomography. J Glaucoma. 2010;19(8):551–5.

64. Mastropasqua R, Fasanella V, Agnifili L, Curcio C, Ciancaglini M, Mastropasqua L. Anterior segment optical coherence tomography imaging of conjunctival filtering blebs after glaucoma surgery. Biomed Res Int. 2014;2014:610623.

65. Sng CCA, Singh M, Chew PTK, et al. Quantitative assessment of changes in trabeculectomy blebs after laser suture lysis using anterior segment coherence tomography. J Glaucoma. 2012;21(5):313–7.

66. Singh M, Aung T, Friedman DS, et al. Anterior segment optical coherence tomography imaging of trabeculectomy blebs before and after laser suture lysis. Am J Ophthalmol. 2007;143(5):873–5.

67. Ichhpujani P, Katz LJ, Gille R, Affel E. Imaging modalities for localization of an iStent ®. Ophthalmic Surg Lasers Imaging. 2010;41(6):660–3.

68. Lenzhofer M, Strohmaier C, Hohensinn M, et al. Longitudinal bleb morphology in anterior segment OCT after minimally invasive transscleral ab interno Glaucoma Gel Microstent implantation. Acta Ophthalmol. 2018;97(2):e231–7.

69. Fuest M, Kuerten D, Koch E, et al. Evaluation of early anatomical changes following canaloplasty with anterior segment spectral-domain optical coherence tomography and ultrasound biomicroscopy. Acta Ophthalmol. 2016;94(5):e287–92.

70. Kuerten D, Plange N, Becker J, Walter P, Fuest M. Evaluation of long-term anatomic changes following Canaloplasty with anterior segment spectral-domain optical coherence tomography and ultrasound biomicroscopy. J Glaucoma. 2018;27(1):87–93.

71. Console JW, Sakata LM, Aung T, Friedman DS, He M. Quantitative analysis of anterior segment optical coherence tomography images: the Zhongshan Angle Assessment Program. Br J Ophthalmol. 2008;92(12):1612–6.

72. Fu H, Xu Y, Lin S, et al. Segmentation and quantification for angle-closure glaucoma assessment in anterior segment oct. IEEE Trans Med Imaging. 2017;36(9):1930–8.

73. Lavanya R, Foster PJ, Sakata LM, et al. Screening for narrow angles in the Singapore population: evaluation of new noncontact screening methods. Ophthalmology. 2008;115(10):1720–7, 1727.e1-2.

74. Xu BY, Burkemper B, Lewinger JP, et al. Correlation between intraocular pressure and angle configuration measured by OCT. Ophthalmol Glaucoma. 2018;1:158–66.

75. Baskaran M, Iyer JV, Narayanaswamy AK, et al. Anterior segment imaging predicts incident gonioscopic angle closure. Ophthalmology. 2015;122(12):2380–4.

Utilizing Optical Coherence Tomography in Glaucoma Management

Timothy P. Fox, Alena Reznik, and Felipe Medeiros

Background

The diagnosis of glaucoma and detection of glaucoma progression are based on structural and functional changes that occur in a characteristic pattern. Functional changes, commonly assessed by standard automated perimetry (SAP), should correlate with optic nerve head (ONH) structure and morphology. Historically, assessment of the ONH and retinal nerve fiber layer (RNFL) was oftentimes subjective with wide variability between examiners and performed by clinical examination and fundus photography [1]. With the advent of optical coherence tomography (OCT) in 1991 [2], evaluation of glaucomatous structural changes has become more objective by allowing for quantifiable and reproducible measurements of the optic nerve head, RNFL, and macular thickness parameters.

T. P. Fox (✉)
Department of Ophthalmology, LAC+USC
Medical Center, Los Angeles, CA, USA
e-mail: tfox@dhs.lacounty.gov

A. Reznik
Southern California Eye Institute, CHA Hollywood
Presbyterian Medical Center, Los Angeles, CA, USA
e-mail: areznik@sceyes.org

F. Medeiros
Clinical Research Unit, Department of
Ophthalmology, Duke University, Durham, NC, USA
e-mail: Felipe.Medeiros@duke.edu

Prior to the development of OCT, confocal scanning laser ophthalmoscopy and scanning laser polarimetry, introduced in the 1980s, were used to assess structural changes in glaucoma. With the development of commercially available Fourier and spectral domain OCT devices (SD-OCT) with improved scan speeds and improved spatial resolution, the use of OCT in glaucoma management has become common practice. Most OCT devices consist of a table-mounted unit that obtains noninvasive, in vivo cross-sectional images of ocular structures and a computer which segments and analyzes the images. Images are obtained by low-coherence interferometry, which measures echo time delay and the magnitude of reflected or backscattered light [3]. Algorithms are utilized to segment structures of interest for further analysis; for instance, the RNFL is measured by detecting the anterior edge of the retinal pigmented epithelium and the photoreceptor layer position to determine the posterior boundary of the RNFL [4].

Early generation OCT machines were based on time domain technology (TD-OCT; e.g., Stratus OCT, Carl Zeiss Meditec, Dublin, CA, USA) which use low-coherence interferometry to obtain two-dimensional images. TD-OCT devices, however, fell out of favor for many clinicians as they were limited by low scan speed (100–400 A scans/second) which resulted in motion artifacts and lower image resolution. More recent commercially available machines

© Springer Nature Switzerland AG 2020
R. Varma et al. (eds.), *Advances in Ocular Imaging in Glaucoma*, Essentials in Ophthalmology,
https://doi.org/10.1007/978-3-030-43847-0_2

are based on spectral-domain (SD-OCT) technology, which has more than 50-fold faster scanning speed as compared with TD-OCT (26,000–53,000 A scans/second), allowing for 1000 A scans to be captured, processed, and displayed within 60 microseconds. The faster image acquisition reduces motion artifacts and results in more stable images. SD-OCT also has improved spatial resolution, providing an axial resolution of 3.9–7 μm—as compared with 8–12 μm with TD-OCT—and transverse resolution of 15–20 μm [5]. Image registration software, available on some devices, minimizes misalignment between consecutive images, improving interscan reproducibility and longitudinal comparison of scans. Studies have demonstrated intraclass correlation between multiple measures of superior, inferior, and average RNFL thickness using SD-OCT in a single individual to be greater than 0.96 [6–8]. The diagnostic accuracy between TD-OCT and SD-OCT has been reported to be either statistically similar [9, 10] or slightly better with SD-OCT [11–17]. Finally, three-dimensional acquisition patterns and advanced segmentation algorithms of SD-OCT devices allow for assessment of macular parameters (Chap. 4). A variety of SD-OCT devices are commercially available, including, but not limited to, Cirrus HD-OCT (Carl Zeiss Meditec, Inc., Dublin, CA, USA), RTVue-100 (Optovue, Inc., Fremont, CA, USA), and Spectralis (Heidelberg Engineering, Dossenheim, Germany). While the information available in this chapter is generalizable to most commercially available SD-OCT devices, it may not be applicable to all.

Diagnosing Glaucoma and Detecting Progression

The use of OCT is a mainstay for the diagnosis of glaucoma and detection of glaucomatous progression. Structural changes in the ONH or RNFL may precede evidence of glaucomatous damage on SAP [18]. Also, some patients with early stage glaucoma may have structural changes alone, referred to as "pre-perimetric" glaucoma [19]. Furthermore, histologic stud-

ies have demonstrated that a significant portion of retinal ganglion cells (RGCs) may be lost before loss is detected on SAP [20]. The use of OCT in glaucoma has primarily focused on assessment of the circumpapillary RNFL (cRNFL) as it allows for comprehensive assessment of all retinal ganglion cells (RGCs) as they approach the ONH.

In SD-OCT, a 6 × 6 mm peripapillary cube consisting of 200 × 200 pixel measurements of a scan data is obtained and segmented to isolate the RNFL. Using high density sampling of the RNFL thickness in this region, a topologic RNFL thickness map is constructed, facilitating examination of the RNFL distribution pattern (Fig. 2.1a, b). Within this map, red encodes thicker and blue encodes thinner RNFL measurements. From the thickness map, an RNFL thickness deviation map is provided. The RNFL thickness deviation map compares the RNFL thickness of the subject to the device's reference database. A pixel is encoded as yellow if the RNFL measurement is below the lower 95% of the centile range for that particular pixel; similarly, pixels are encoded red if below the lower 99% of the centile range [21].

CRNFL thickness is measured at a circle 3.46 mm in diameter (1.76 mm radius) centered on the optic disc. Although this fixed distance is somewhat arbitrary, this scan circle size was found to higher reproducibility than measurements from with other circle diameters [22]. While this fixed distance may allow for more reproducible cRNFL measures, RNFL defects existing outside of this area may be missed. The average or global cRNFL is provided along with the thickness of inferior, superior, nasal, and temporal quadrants. Quadrants are further broken down to clock hours in a similar fashion (Fig. 2.1a, b). These measures are compared to age-matched controls based on a reference database, which varies based on the machine used. Colors are utilized to denote normal from abnormal measurements based on the reference database. Green encodes a thickness measurement within normal distribution or within two standard deviations of the average reference population; yellow, a thickness measurement <5% of the population; red, a thickness measurement <1% of

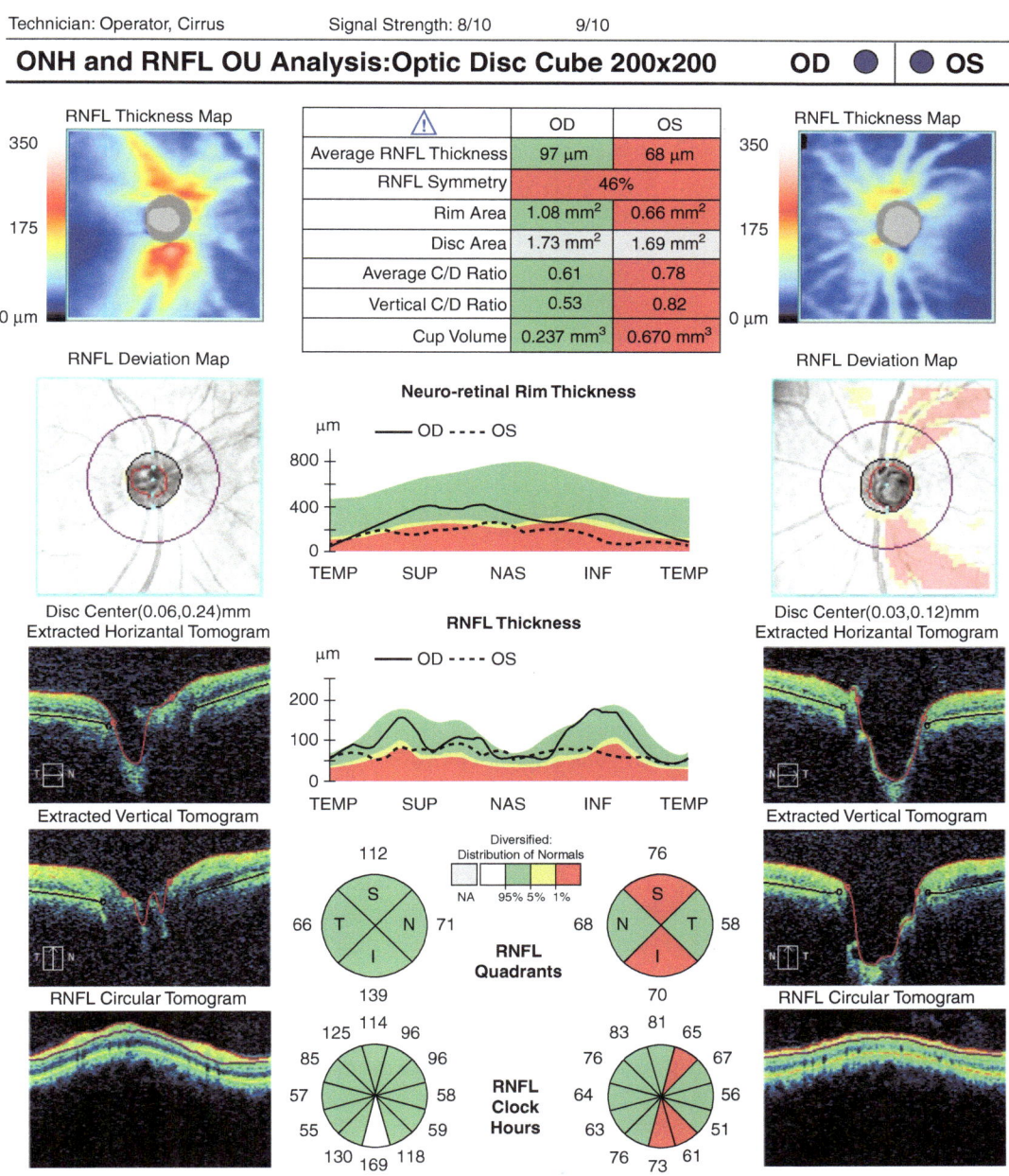

Fig. 2.1 (**a**) Cirrus HD-OCT RNFL thickness map of the right eye demonstrating robust RNFL arcuate bundles. No defects are detected on the RNFL deviation map. Average RNFL thickness, rim area, average C/D ratio, vertical C/D ratio, and cup volume are within normal distribution as compared with age-matched controls within the reference population. Sectoral analysis is also within normal distribution. (**b**) The same patient's left eye, which demonstrates RNFL thinning and attenuation on the thickness map, noted by the paucity of orange and red along the normal RNFL arcuate distribution. On the RNFL deviation map, clear inferotemporal and superotemporal RNFL defects are noted in wedge-shaped distributions. Average RNFL thickness, RNFL symmetry between the eyes, rim area, average C/D ratio, vertical C/D, and cup volume are all below 1% of age-matched controls within the reference population. Sectoral analysis also confirms relative thinning of the superior and inferior quadrants below 1% of the average reference population

the population; and white, a thickness measurement >5% of the population.

The pattern of RNFL loss on OCT mirrors neuroretinal rim thinning. RNFL thickness generally follows the "ISNT" rule—that is, RNFL is thickest inferiorly followed by superiorly, nasally, and temporally—and violation of this rule may indicate glaucoma. The inferior RNFL quadrant typically undergoes the greatest amount of thinning; it also has the greatest area under the receiver operating characteristics curve valve (AUC) for detection of glaucoma [11]. The nasal and temporal quadrants generally have a low AUC, particularly in early glaucoma, and thinning in these quadrants may indicate the presence of a non-glaucomatous optic neuropathy.

The diagnostic ability of SD-OCT to discriminate between glaucomatous and healthy eyes has an AUC of approximately 0.9, though several factors have an effect on diagnostic abilities, including glaucoma severity [23]. SD-OCT has also been shown to discriminate between eyes with preperimetric glaucoma—defined as eyes with progression on follow-up optic disc stereoscopic photographs but without visual field defect during the study's 5 year follow-up period—and those with suspected glaucoma, with an AUC of 0.86 [24].

To recognize glaucoma progression, it is important to understand the interscan reproducibility and variability of SD-OCT. Intraclass correlation coefficients of global cRNFL thickness are excellent with an intravisit value of 0.986 and intervisit value of 0.972 [6]. These intravisit and intervisit correlation values are better with SD-OCT compared to TD-OCT. The intervisit tolerance limit for global cRNFL thickness is 3.89 μm, which is often rounded to 4 μm. Because of the intervisit variability, examiners should consider at least 8 μm, or twice the standard deviation value, to be a clinically significant change in RNFL thickness.

When assessing for progression, it is important to assess not only for overall change but also for focal change. The RNFL thickness map facilitates analysis of these defects and patterns of progression. Three common glaucomatous patterns may occur, including a new RNFL defect, widening of an existing defect or deepening of an existing defect without widening. The most common area of progressive RNFL thinning is located inferotemporally. Conventional sectoral or global analysis may overlook localized defects or focal areas of progression as focal defects may be masked when averaging cRNFL thickness (Fig. 2.2). RNFL progression was found to most commonly occur at 2 mm from the disc center [21], further away from the optic disc center than the 1.76 mm radius where cRNFL is measured. It is important, therefore, to examine the RNFL thickness and deviation maps, which may reveal focal changes. Focusing on these localized changes, referred to as the region of interest, has been shown to be superior to global RNFL thickness [25]. Whenever progression is suspected, confirmatory testing should be performed.

Two basic strategies, event-based and trend-based analyses, are employed when assessing for glaucoma progression. Event-based analysis compares one test to another, and progression is determined when change occurs below a preset threshold as compared with baseline. As previously noted, there can be up to approximately 4 μm of intervisit variability with SD-OCT, and progression should be strongly suspected when there is a difference of 8 μm or greater between tests. One should also compare the current test to baseline tests, which should ideally be two reliable and stable tests done within a limited time period early in the patient's clinical course. Event-based analysis has various limitations, and it may falsely identify progression if the test in question is unreliable. It is also susceptible to outlier results. If comparing scans five or more years apart, it is important to account for normal aging. Cross-sectional analysis has shown a negative correlation between age and average RNFL thickness of −0.33 μm/year while longitudinal analysis reported a change of −0.52 μm/year [14, 26].

RNFL Thickness Map

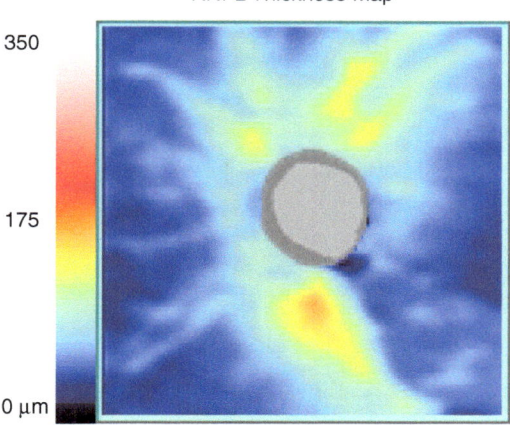

350

175

0 μm

RNFL Deviation Map

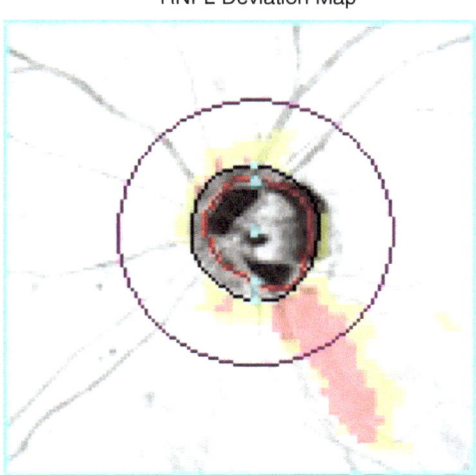

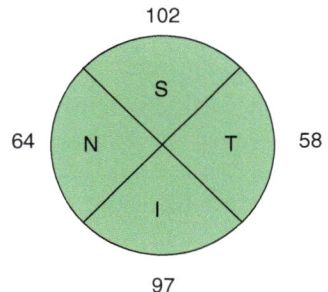

102

S

64   N   T   58

I

97

Fig. 2.2 Cirrus HD-OCT RNFL deviation map demonstrating focal inferotemporal thinning which is not detected by sectoral analysis or average RNFL thickness, both of which are within normal distribution as compared with age-matched controls of the average reference population

Trend-based analysis evaluates a series of at least four sequential tests, including baseline tests, and measures the slope of change over time [27]. Trend-based analysis is performed by change analysis software, first available in the third generation of TD-OCT devices (Stratus OCT) as Guided Progression Analysis (GPA). Many currently commercially available SD-OCT devices include change analysis software, and it has been shown to be useful in both determining glaucoma progression and the rate of progression. Progression is detected when there is a significant negative slope of the regression line, and the slope of the regression line represents the rate of RNFL thinning, expressed in micrometers per year (Fig. 2.3). Change analysis can be performed not only with global cRNFL thickness but also sectors. Trend-based analysis is less susceptible to fluctuation and outlier results, and it takes into account normal age-related RNFL thinning through linear regression analysis. The regression line slope is also useful in estimating the rate of disease progression. Trend-based analysis, however, requires a large number of tests. Therefore, this type of analysis is less sensitive to sudden and dramatic changes in RNFL thickness.

The rate of change for average cRNFL thickness in patients with glaucoma progression ranges widely, from -0.72 μm/year to -15.4 μm/year as determined by prospective studies [27, 28]. SD-OCT (Cirrus HD-OCT) appears to be superior to TD-OCT (Stratus OCT) for the detection of progression using trend analysis software and cRNFL thickness [29]. GPA may also be used to detect progression based on the RNFL thickness map, though this is currently available only with Cirrus HD-OCT devices. This is performed through computing differences in RNFL thickness change map between two baseline measurements and a follow-up image for each of the individual 50×50 superpixels (one superpixel is equivalent to 4×4 pixels) contained in the 6×6 mm RNFL thickness map. Superpixels are encoded yellow on the RNFL thickness change map if the difference is greater than the test-retest

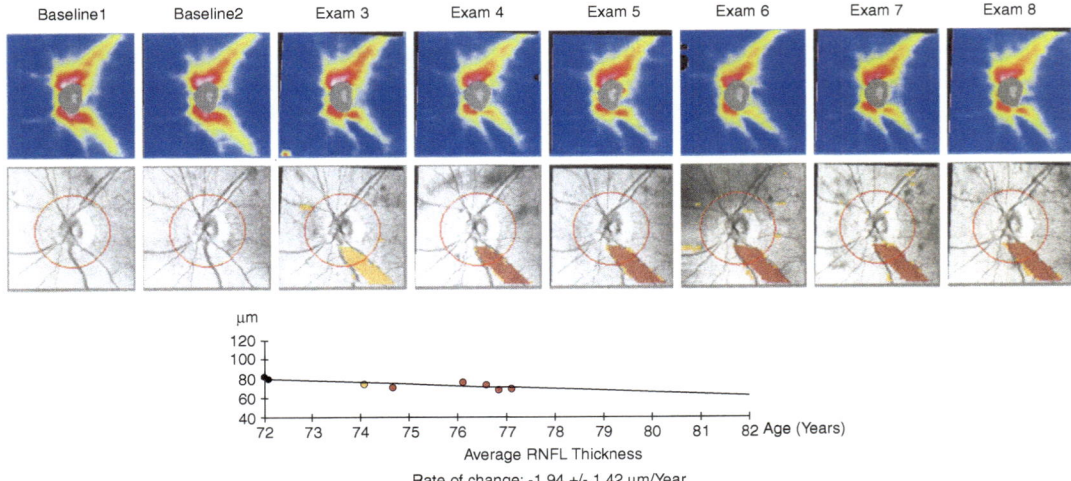

Fig. 2.3 Guided progression analysis demonstrating glaucoma progression of the left eye. By Exam 3, possible progression was detected, noted by the yellow inferior sector on the deviation map. Progression was subsequently confirmed by Exam 4, noted by the change in color to red on the deviation map

probability. Once this difference is confirmed on subsequent testing, the superpixel is encoded in red. The GPA analysis thickness map displays these colors when at least 20 contiguous pixels demonstrate significant change [5] (Fig. 2.3).

OCT also provides a variety of optic nerve head parameters [30], including rim area, cup area, and cup-to-disc ratio (Fig. 2.1a, b). While the agreement between neuroretinal rim and RNFL measurements was poor in the detection of glaucoma progression when utilizing TD-OCT [31], the improved resolution of optic disc images in SD-OCT makes optic nerve head parameters useful in the diagnosis of glaucoma and detecting glaucomatous progression [32]. The vertical rim thickness, vertical cup-to-disc ratio, cup-to-disc ratio, and horizontal rim thickness have been shown to outperform other optic nerve head parameters in distinguishing normal eyes from glaucomatous eyes of all severities, with AUC ranging from 0.901 to 0.963. In discriminating between normal eyes and eyes with mild glaucoma, vertical cup-to-disc ratio, rim area, and vertical rim thickness have been shown to be of most benefit [33]. The low reproducibility of optic nerve head scans and misidentification of the optic disc or cup margin have led to many clinicians preferring RNFL measures over optic nerve head parameters for the diagnosis of glaucoma; however, it is important to note that misidentification of the optic nerve tissue may be manually corrected.

SD-OCT also allows for visualization of Bruch's membrane opening (BMO) for enhanced examination of the neuroretinal rim and improved detection of glaucoma. Evaluating BMO is important, as the clinically visible disc margin seen on fundoscopy does not correspond to a consistent anatomic structure on OCT. Studies suggest utilizing Bruch's membrane opening-minimum rim width (BMO-MRW), defined as the width between the termination of Bruch's membrane, as the anatomic border of the optic disc margin, which has improved diagnostic performance as compared with confocal scanning laser tomography, which measures the perceived disc margin without reference to the rim tissue orientation [34].

Pitfalls of Interpreting Results

The ability of OCT devices to discriminate between healthy and glaucomatous eyes and to detect progression is limited by the quality of the reference databases. The reference databases are based on age-matched healthy controls and are not transferrable between devices. The Cirrus HD-OCT database includes 284 non-glaucomatous subjects from seven study sites, of which six were from the USA and one from China. Forty-three percent were Caucasian, 24% Asian, 18% African descent, 12% Hispanic, and 1% Indian, and 6% were unspecified or mixed. The subjects ranged from 18 to 84 years of age and had refractive errors between −12.00 diopters and +8.00 diopters, but few subjects had refractive errors on the extreme sides of the spectrum. Subjects were excluded if they had visual field loss, an RNFL defect, disc hemorrhage, or IOP >21 mm Hg [35]. The RTVue version 4.0 software database includes 861 healthy eyes from 15 clinical sites, including six from the USA, one from England, three from China, three from Japan, and two from India. Subjects ranged from 19 to 82 years of age and had normal visual fields and IOP <22 mm Hg. Twenty-nine percent of subjects were Chinese, 19% Japanese, 18% Caucasian, 14% Indian, and 11% Hispanic, and 9% were of African descent [36]. The Spectralis

SD-OCT database includes data from 201 healthy subjects from one study site in Germany. All subjects were Caucasian, ranging from ages 18 to 78. Subjects were excluded if they had a family history of glaucoma, IOP >21 mmHg, evidence of visual field damage or refractive error worse than −7 diopters [37].

Several factors can affect OCT measurements and potentially lead to misinterpretation and misdiagnosis and should be considered when analyzing scan results. These factors include signal strength, signal blocking, segmentation error, age, race/ethnicity, refractive error, optic disc size, and glaucoma severity [38]. Signal strength can affect OCT measurements, as lower signal strengths underestimate RNFL thickness, resulting in falsely thin RNFL measurements, particularly in myopic eyes. Signal strength may be affected by many variables, including dry eye, corneal edema, cataract, media opacities, and vitreous floaters. It has been suggested, at least with Stratus TD-OCT, that examiners aim for a signal strength of at least seven [39]. It is important to take signal strength into account, particularly as signal strength may decrease over time as patients develop media opacities (Figs. 2.4 and 2.5). It has also been

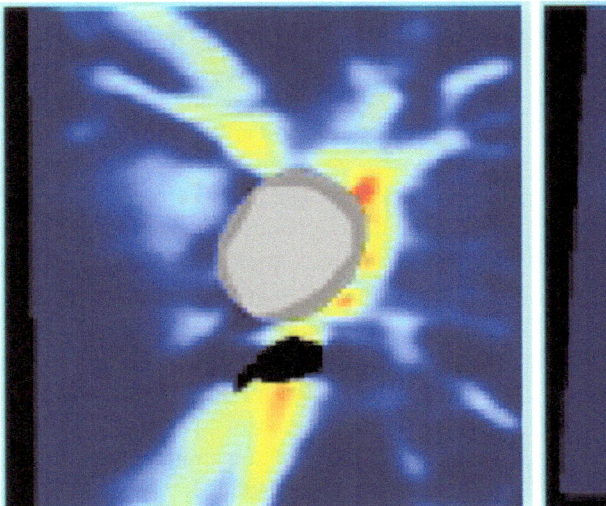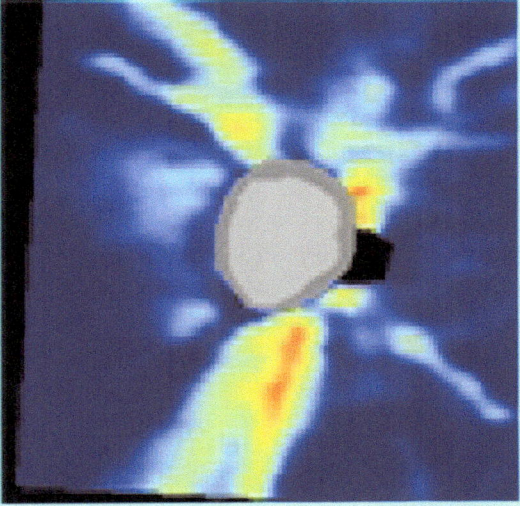

Fig. 2.4 Cirrus HD-OCT of the right eye demonstrating signal blockage from a PVD. Follow-up examination demonstrates movement of the vitreous opacity

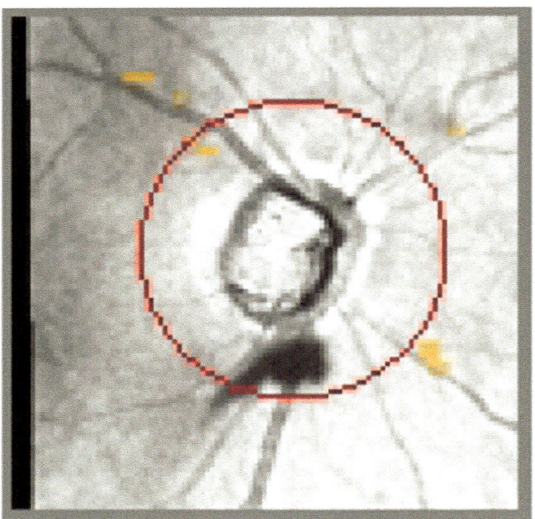 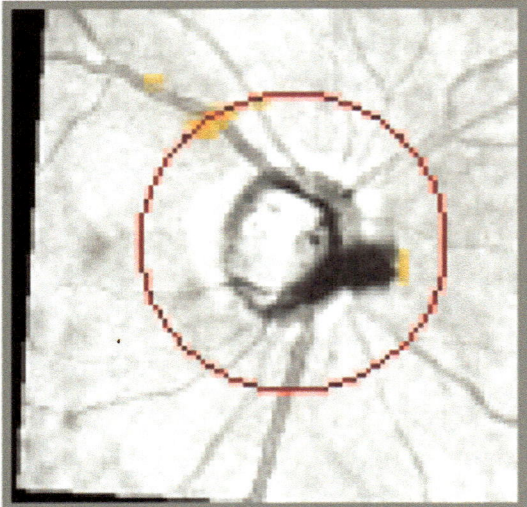

Fig. 2.4 (continued)

shown that multifocal lenses may affect scan quality, leading to wavy horizontal artifacts [40].

OCT measurements are also subject to segmentation errors. Current SD-OCT devices utilize automated segmentation to define the ONH and various structures of interest; however, this may inaccurately identify intraocular structures. Relying on automated segmentation without manual refinement has been shown to reduce global cRNFL thickness and overestimate the diagnosis of glaucoma, particularly in eyes with thinner RNFLs, scans with lower signal strength, and patients of older age. Operators should inspect scans for aberrant segmentation and if identified should manually refine the segmentation [41].

Refractive errors, most notably myopia, may affect RNFL measurements. While myopia is a risk factor for the development of glaucoma, it may also lead to erroneously thin cRNFL and macular thickness measurements due to optical projection artifact of the scanning area. Non-glaucomatous myopic eyes may be incorrectly classified as abnormal by OCT analysis due to limited reference database [42]. As previously mentioned, reference databases only included refractive errors between −12.00 and +8.00 diopters, with few patients on the extreme ends of the refractive error spectrum. Moderately and highly myopic eyes have thinner global cRNFL and thinner superior and inferior quadrants [43–45]. Interestingly, non-glaucomatous myopic eyes tend to have thicker temporal cRNFL quadrants [46]. This may be due, in part, to the effect of myopia on the RNFL distribution pattern. With increasing myopia, the superotemporal and inferotemporal RNFL bundles tend to converge temporally [47].

As previously mentioned, there is a normal rate of RNFL thinning that occurs with age, ranging from −0.33 to −0.52 µm/year of RNFL loss. While age is taken into account with trend-based analysis, also remember to account for age-related loss with event-based analysis, particularly if the studies are 5 years or more apart [27]. Race and ethnicity appear to also have an effect on OCT measurements and analysis. Clinicians should be cautious when interpreting data of non-Caucasian patients, particularly those of African or Asian ancestry [48]. Differences seen may be in part due to limited reference databases. It has been found that patients of African ancestry have the thinnest temporal quadrant, corresponding with thinner papillomacular RNFL bundles, and thicker measurements in inferior and superior regions [35, 49]. It has been suggested that Asians may have thicker global, superior, and inferior cRNFL thickness values and Hispanics may have

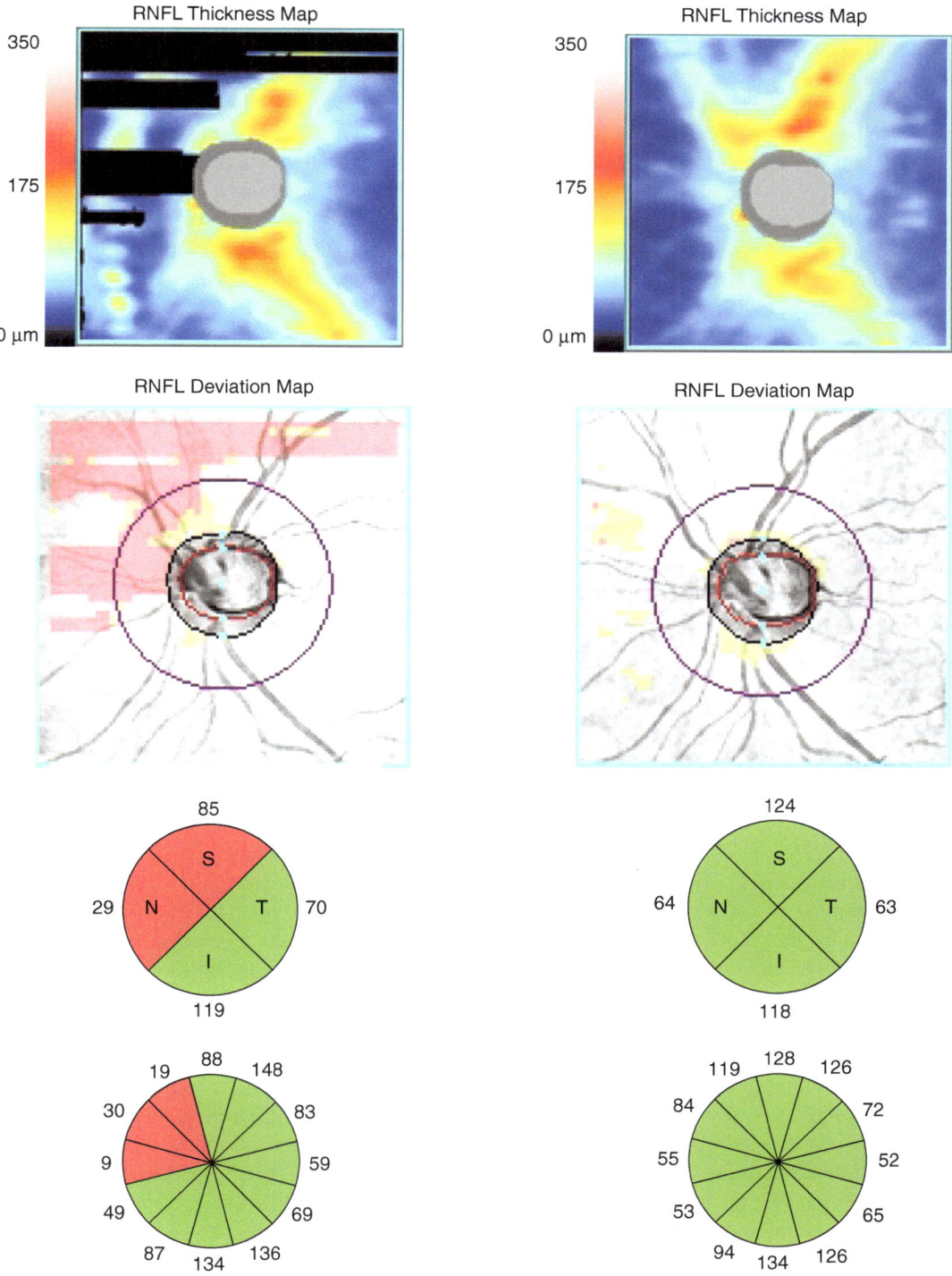

Fig. 2.5 Cirrus HD-OCT of the left eye demonstrating significant signal dropout superiorly and nasally, causing artifactual thinning on sectoral analysis. Repeat scan of the left eye without signal dropout, demonstrating a full RNFL without thinning on sectoral analysis

thicker global and inferior cRNFL thickness values [50]. The differences may be in part due to large ONH in Hispanic patients or those with African or Asian ancestry [51]. A correlation has also been demonstrated between longer axial lengths and thinner temporal RNFL quadrants in patients with Asian ancestry [45, 52].

Optic disc size may also have an effect on OCT measurements and analysis. Larger optic discs, particularly those greater than 2 mm in diameter, may have falsely thicker RNFL values. This is because cRNFL thickness is greater closer to the disc, and most OCT devices measure cRNFL thickness at a set 3.4 mm radius away from the disc center. In these patients, RNFL topography may be a better measure to assess for thinning.

Finally, glaucoma severity may have an effect on OCT measurements and performance. When diagnosing patients with glaucoma, SD-OCT has been found to have improved AUC and sensitivities and specificities with decreasing SAP visual field index values [53]. There is also improved ability of SD-OCT to discriminate between healthy eyes and those with advanced disease as compared with discrimination between eyes with early stage glaucoma [54]. By similar accord, the rate of RNFL loss is associated with the baseline RNFL thickness, with thicker baseline RNFL being associated with a faster rate of RNFL loss [27].

The utility of OCT in detecting glaucoma progression in patients with severe glaucoma is limited by the "floor effect." "Floor" refers to the cRNFL architectural support made up of blood vessels and retinal glial cells, such as Müller cells, astroglia, and microglia, which do not degenerate with retinal ganglion cell axons. As the RNFL thins, the contribution of these supportive structures is more substantive, rendering OCT less sensitive in identifying and segmenting the RNFL in advanced glaucoma (Fig. 2.6). The average cRNFL thickness rarely drops below 50–60 μm, and never below 30 μm, even in eyes with no-light perception vision [55]. The "floor" value varies with different SD-OCT devices and was found to be an average 57 μm on Cirrus HD-OCT, 64.7 μm with RTVue, and 49.2 μm with Spectralis SD-OCT. The RNFL "floor"

is reached around relative SAP sensitivities between −11.3 and −14.4 dB and RNFL thinning stops around sensitivities between −19.3 and −23.7 dB [56]. Because of this, RNFL measurements by OCT are less sensitive than SAP in the detection of progression in advanced glaucoma. Macular measurements, discussed separately, may provide an alternative way to objectively and quantitatively assess for structural progression in advanced glaucoma.

Future Uses of SD-OCT

As with most testing for glaucoma, the use of one single parameter on OCT may misdiagnose healthy eyes as having glaucoma or glaucomatous eyes as being healthy. Recent evidence suggests combining more than one individual OCT parameter, such as ONH measurements, RNFL, or macular measurements, may be advantageous in reducing these diagnostic errors. The Glaucoma Structural Diagnostic Index, or GSDI, found that combining these OCT parameters is significantly better than the single best parameter [57].

Researchers have also evaluated the relationship between structural and functional damage in the diagnosis, staging, and monitoring of glaucoma, potentially providing insight on how visual function behaves relative to structural damage [58]. Various models have been proposed to examine this relationship. Common visual field maps utilized include the Garway-Heath structure function map and Kanamori visual field cluster map [59, 60].

Because loss of RGCs are the primary underlying pathologic feature in glaucoma, various models have been proposed to estimate the number of RGCs based on OCT RNFL thickness measures [61]. Recently, the combined structure-function index (CSFI) has been proposed to estimate the percentage of RGCs lost as compared to healthy age-matched controls. The CSFI combines structural and functional test results into an index to aid examiners in diagnosing and prognosticating glaucomatous eyes. The CSFI has been shown to be superior to SD-OCT RNFL thickness alone in discriminating glaucomatous from normal

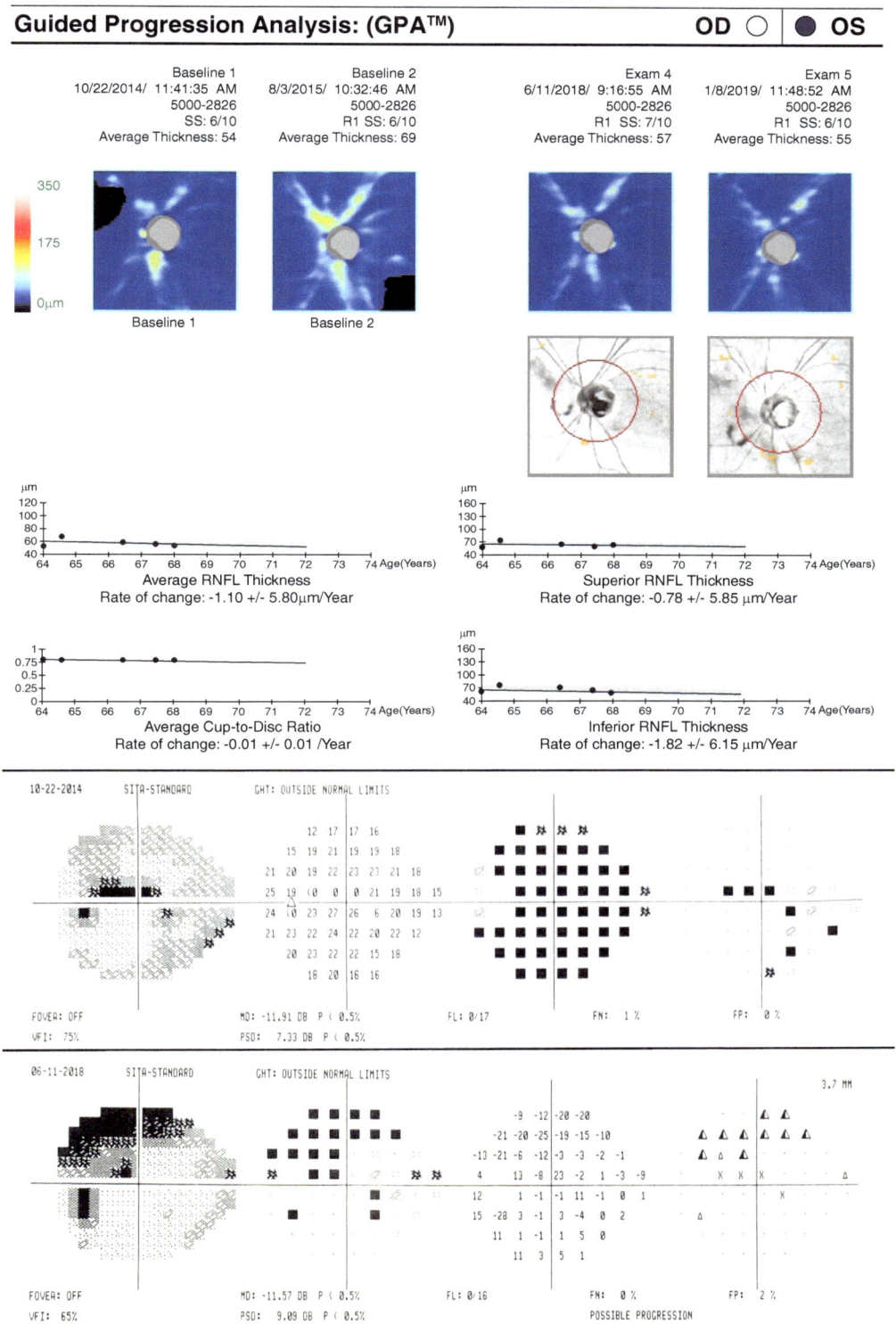

Fig. 2.6 Cirrus HD-OCT GPA demonstrating stable RNFL thickness in advanced glaucoma, likely at or near the floor. During the same time period, patient had possible progression on standard automated perimetry

eyes, with an AUC of 0.94, and a similar ability as SD-OCT to discriminate between healthy and preperimetric glaucoma eyes [62]. Because SAP abnormalities may occasionally precede detection of structural loss, the CSFI may have advantages over SD-OCT alone as it utilizes the strengths of both structural and functional testing. With the advent of a newer generation OCT device called swept-source OCT, direct visualization and segmentation of the RGC layer has been possible [63]. These newer technologies may increase our understanding of the structure-function relationship in glaucoma and may aid in earlier detection of glaucoma and its progression.

Compliance with Ethical Requirements Fox, Alena Reznik, and Felipe Medeiros declare they have no conflict of interest. No human or animal studies were carried out by the authors for this article.

References

1. Lichter PR. Variability of expert observers in evaluating the optic disc. Trans Am Ophthalmol Soc. 1976;74:532–72.
2. Huang D, Swanson EA, Lin CP, et al. Optical coherence tomography. Science. 1991;254:1178–81.
3. Srinivasan RJ, Wojtkowski M, Witkin AJ, et al. High-definition and 3-dimensional imaging of macular pathologies with high-speed ultrahigh-resolution optical coherence tomography. Ophthalmology. 2006;113:2054.e1–14. https://doi.org/10.1016/j.ophtha.2006.05.046.
4. Trick GL, Calotti FY, Skarf B. Advances in imaging of the optic disc and retinal nerve fiber layer. J Neuroophthalmol. 2006;26(4):284–95. https://doi.org/10.1097/01.wno.0000249327.65227.67.
5. Leung CK. Diagnosing glaucoma progression with optical coherence tomography. Curr Opin Ophthalmol. 2014;25(2):104–11. https://doi.org/10.1097/ICU.0000000000000024.
6. Mwanza JC, Chang RT, Budenz DL, et al. Reproducibility of peripapillary retinal nerve fiber layer thickness and optic nerve head parameters measured with Cirrus HD-OCT in glaucomatous eyes. Invest Ophthalmol Vis Sci. 2010;51:5724–30. https://doi.org/10.1167/iovs.10-5222.
7. Garas A, Vargha P, Hollo G. Reproducibility of retinal nerve fiber layer and macular thickness measurement with the RTVue-100 optical coherence tomograph. Ophthalmology. 2010;117:738–46. https://doi.org/10.1016/j.ophtha.2009.08.039.
8. Menke MN, Knecht P, Sturm V, et al. Reproducibility of nerve fiber layer thickness measurements using 3D fourier-domain OCT. Invest Ophthalmol Vis Sci. 2008;49:5386–91. https://doi.org/10.1167/iovs.07-1435.
9. Wong JJ, Chen TC, Shen LQ, et al. Macular imaging for glaucoma using spectral-domain optical coherence tomography: a review. Semin Ophthalmol. 2012;27:160–6. https://doi.org/10.3109/08820538.2012.712734.
10. Mansouri K, Leite MT, Medeiros FA, et al. Assessment of rates of structural change in glaucoma using imaging technologies. Eye. 2011;25:269–77. https://doi.org/10.1038/eye.2010.202.
11. Leung CK-S, Cheung CY-L, Weinreb RN, et al. Retinal nerve fiber layer imaging with spectral-domain optical coherence tomography: a variability and diagnostic performance study. Ophthalmology. 2009;116(7):1257–63. https://doi.org/10.1016/j.ophtha.2009.04.013.
12. Sung KR, Kim DY, Park SB, Kook MS. Comparison of retinal nerve fiber layer thickness measured by cirrus HD and Stratus optical coherence tomography. Ophthalmology. 2009;116(7):1264–70. https://doi.org/10.1016/j.ophtha.2008.12.045.
13. Chang RT, Knight OJ, Feuer WJ, Budenz DL. Sensitivity and specificity of time-domain versus spectral-domain optical coherence tomography in diagnosing early to moderate glaucoma. Ophthalmology. 2009;116(12):2294–9. https://doi.org/10.1016/j.ophtha.2009.06.012.
14. Knight OJ, Chang RT, Feuer WJ, Budenz DL. Comparison of retinal nerve fiber layer measurements using time domain and spectral domain optical coherent tomography. Ophthalmology. 2009;116(7):1271–7. https://doi.org/10.1016/j.ophtha.2008.12.032.
15. Vizzeri G, Weinreb RN, Gonzalez-Garcia AO, et al. Agreement between spectral-domain and time-domain OCT for measuring RNFL thickness. Br J Ophthalmol. 2009;93(6):775–81. https://doi.org/10.1136/bjo.2008.150698.
16. Jeoung JW, Park KH, Kim TW, et al. Diagnostic ability of optical coherence tomography with a normative database to detect localized retinal nerve fiber layer defects. Ophthalmology. 2005;112(12):2157–63. https://doi.org/10.1016/j.ophtha.2005.07.012.
17. Moreno-Montañés J, Olmo N, Alvarez A, et al. Cirrus high-definition optical coherence tomography compared with stratus optical coherence tomography in glaucoma diagnosis. Invest Ophtalmol Vis Sci. 2010;51(1):335–43. https://doi.org/10.1167/iovs.08-2988.
18. Sommer A, Katz J, Quigley HA, et al. Clinically detectable nerve fiber atrophy precedes the onset of glaucomatous field loss. Arch Ophthalmol. 1991;109(1):77–83.
19. Zhang X, Dastiridou A, Francis BA, et al. Comparison of glaucoma progression detection by optical coherence tomography and visual field.

Am J Ophthalmol. 2017;184:63–74. https://doi.org/10.1016/j.ajo.2017.09.020.

20. Kerrigan-Baumrind LA, Quigley HA, Pease ME, et al. Number of ganglion cells in glaucoma eyes compared with threshold visual field tests in the same persons. Invest Ophthalmol Vis Sci. 2000;41(3):741–8.

21. Leung CK, Yu M, Weinreb RN. Retinal nerve fiber layer imaging with spectral-domain optical coherence tomography: patterns of retinal nerve fiber layer progression. Ophthalmology. 2012;119(9):1858–66. https://doi.org/10.1016/j.ophtha.2012.03.044.

22. Schuman JS, Pedut-Kloizman T, Hertzmark E, et al. Reproducibility of nerve fiber layer thickness measurements using optical coherence tomography. Ophthalmology. 1996;103(11):1889–98.

23. Bussel II, Wolstein G, Schuman JS. OCT for glaucoma diagnosis, screening and detection of glaucoma progression. Br J Ophthalmol. 2014;98(Suppl 2):ii15–9. https://doi.org/10.1136/bjophthalmol-2013-304326.

24. Lisboa R, Leite MT, Zangwill LM, et al. Diagnosing preperimetric glaucoma with spectral domain optical coherence tomography. Ophthalmology. 2012;119(11):2261–9. https://doi.org/10.1016/j.ophtha.2012.06.009.

25. Hood DC, Xin D, Wang D, et al. A region-of-interest approach for detecting progression of glaucomatous damage with optical coherence tomography. JAMA Ophthalmol. 2015;133(12):1438–44. https://doi.org/10.1001/jamaophthalmol.2015.3871.

26. Leung CK, Yu M, Weinreb RN, et al. Retinal nerve fiber layer imaging with spectral-domain optical coherence tomography: a prospective analysis of age-related loss. Ophthalmology. 2012;119(4):731–7. https://doi.org/10.1016/j.ophtha.2011.10.010.

27. Leung CK, Cheung CY, Weinreb RN, et al. Evaluation of retinal nerve fiber layer progression in glaucoma: a study on optical coherence tomography guided progression analysis. Invest Ophthalmol Vis Sci. 2010;51(1):217–22. https://doi.org/10.1167/iovs.09-3468.

28. Medeiros FA, Zangwill LM, Alencar LM, et al. Detection of glaucoma progression with stratus OCT retinal nerve fiber layer, optic nerve head, and macular thickness measurements. Invest Ophthalmol Vis Sci. 2009;50(12):5741–8. https://doi.org/10.1167/iovs.09-3715.

29. Leung CK, Chiu V, Weinreb RN, et al. Evaluation of retinal nerve fiber layer progression in glaucoma: a comparison between spectral-domain and time-domain optical coherence tomography. Ophthalmology. 2011;118(8):1558–62. https://doi.org/10.1016/j.ophtha.2011.01.026.

30. Mwanza J-C, Oakley JD, Budenz DL, et al. Ability of the Cirrus HD-OCT optic nerve head parameters to discriminate normal from glaucomatous eyes. Ophthalmology. 2011;118:241–8.

31. Leung CK, Liu S, Weinreb RN, et al. Evaluation of retinal nerve fiber layer progression in glaucoma: a prospective analysis with neuroretinal rim and visual field progression. Ophthalmology. 2011;118(8):1551–7. https://doi.org/10.1016/j.ophtha.2010.12.035.

32. Naghizadeh F, Garas A, Vargha P, et al. Detection of early glaucomatous progression with different parameters of the RTVue optical coherence tomography. J Glaucoma. 2014;23(4):195–8. https://doi.org/10.1097/IJG.0b013e31826a9707.

33. Na JH, Sung KR, Lee JR, et al. Detection of glaucomatous progression by spectral-domain optical coherence tomography. Ophthalmology. 2013;120(7):1388–95. https://doi.org/10.1016/j.ophtha.2012.12.014.

34. Chauhan BC, O'Leary N, Almobarak FA, et al. Enhanced detection of open-angle glaucoma with an anatomically accurate optical coherence tomography-derived neuroretinal rim parameter. Ophthalmology. 2013;120(3):535–43. https://doi.org/10.1016/j.ophtha.2012.09.055.

35. Knight OJ, Girkin CA, Budenz DL, et al. Cirrus OCT Normative Database Study Group. Effect of race, age, and axial length on optic nerve head parameters and retinal nerve fiber layer thickness measured by Cirrus HD-OCT. Arch Ophthalmol. 2012;130(3):312–8. https://doi.org/10.1001/archopthalmol.2011.1576.

36. Sinai MJ, Garway-Heath DF, Fingeret M, et al. The role of ethnicity on the retinal nerve fiber layer and optic disc area measured with Fourier domain optical coherence tomography. Invest Ophthalmol Vis Sci. 2009;50((13):abstract 4785.

37. Silverman AL, Hammel N, Khachatryan N, et al. Diagnostic accuracy of the Spectralis and cirrus reference database in differentiating between healthy and early glaucoma eyes. Ophthalmology. 2016;123(2):408–14. https://doi.org/10.1016/j.ophtha.2015.09.047.

38. Chong GT, Lee RK. Glaucoma versus red disease: imaging and glaucoma diagnosis. Curr Opin Ophthalmol. 2012;23(2):79–88. https://doi.org/10.1097/ICU.0b013e32834ff431.

39. Wu Z, Huang J, Dustin L, Sadda SR. Signal strength is an important determinant of accuracy of nerve fiber layer thickness measurement by optical coherence tomography. J Glaucoma. 2009;18(3):213–6. https://doi.org/10.1097/IJG.0b013e31817eee20.

40. Inoue M, Bissen-Miyajima H, Yoshino M, Suzuki T. Wavy horizontal artifacts on optical coherence tomography line-scanning images caused by diffractive multifocal intraocular lenses. J Cataract Refract Surg. 2009;35:1239–43. https://doi.org/10.1016/j.jcrs.2009.04.016.

41. Mansberger SL, Menda SA, Fortune BA, et al. Automated segmentation errors when using optical coherence tomography to measure retinal nerve fiber layer thickness in glaucoma. Am J Ophthalmol. 2017;174:1–8. https://doi.org/10.1016/j.ajo.2016.10.020.

42. Mwanza JC, Sayyad FE, Aref AA, et al. Rates of abnormal retinal nerve fiber layer and ganglion cell layer OCT scans in healthy myopic eyes: cirrus versus RTVue. Ophthalmic Surg Lasers

Imaging. 2012;43(6 Suppl):S67–74. https://doi.org/10.3928/15428877-20121003-01.

43. Rauscher FM, Sekhon N, Feuer WJ, Budenz DL. Myopia affects retinal nerve fiber layer measurements as determined by optical coherence tomography. J Glaucoma. 2009;18(7):501–5. https://doi.org/10.1097/IJG.0b013e318193c2be.

44. Leung CK, Mohamed S, Leung KS, et al. Retinal nerve fiber layer measurements in myopia: an optical coherence tomography study. Invest Ophthalmol Vis Sci. 2006;47(12):5171–6.

45. Kang SH, Hong SW, Im SK, et al. Effect of myopia on the thickness of the retinal nerve fiber layer measured by Cirrus HD optical coherence tomography. Invest Ophthalmol Vis Sci. 2010;51(8):4075–83. https://doi.org/10.1167/iovs.09-4737.

46. Akashi A, Kanamori A, Ueda K, et al. The ability of SD-OCT to differentiate early glaucoma with high myopia from highly myopic controls and non-highly myopic controls. Invest Ophthalmol Vis Sci. 2015;56(11):6573–80. https://doi.org/10.1167/iovs.15-17635.

47. Leung CK, Yu M, Weinreb RN, et al. Retinal nerve fiber layer imaging with spectral-domain optical coherence tomography: interpreting the RNFL maps in healthy myopic eyes. Invest Ophthalmol Vis Sci. 2012;53:7194–200. https://doi.org/10.1167/iovs.12-9726.

48. Budenz DL, Anderson DR, Varma R, et al. Determinants of normal retinal nerve fiber layer thickness measured by Stratus OCT. Ophthalmology. 2007;114(6):1046–52. https://doi.org/10.1016/j.ophtha.2006.08.046.

49. Girkin CA, Sample PA, Liebmann JM et al; ADAGES Group. African Descent and Glaucoma Evaluation Study (ADAGES), II: ancestry differences in optic disc, retinal nerve fiber layer, and macular structure in healthy subjects. Arch Ophthalmol. 2010;128(5):541–550. https://doi.org/10.1001/archophthalmol.2010.49.

50. Poon LY, Antar H, Tsikata E, et al. Effects of age, race, and ethnicity on the optic nerve and peripapillary region using spectral-domain OCT 3D volume scans. Transl Vis Sci Technol. 2018;7(6):12. https://doi.org/10.1167/tvst.7.6.12.

51. Seider MI, Lee RY, Wang D, et al. Optic disk size variability between African, Asian, white, Hispanic, and Filipino Americans using Heidelberg retinal tomography. J Glaucoma. 2009;18(8):595–600. https://doi.org/10.1097/IJG.0b013e3181996f05.

52. Kim MJ, Lee EJ, Kim TW. Peripapillary retinal nerve fibre layer thickness profile in subjects with myopia measured using the Stratus optical coherence tomography. Br J Ophthalmol. 2010;94(1):115–20. https://doi.org/10.1136/bjo.2009.162206.

53. Leite MT, Zangwill LM, Weinreb RN, et al. Effect of disease severity on the performance of Cirrus spectral-domain OCT for glaucoma diagnosis. Invest Ophthalmol Vis Sci. 2010;51(8):4104–9. https://doi.org/10.1167/iovs.09-4716.

54. Bengtsson B, Andersson S, Heijl A. Performance of time-domain and spectral-domain Optical Coherence Tomography for glaucoma screening. Acta Ophthalmol. 2010;90(4):310–5.

55. Chan CK, Miller NR. Peripapillary nerve fiber layer thickness measured by optical coherence tomography in patients with no light perception from long-standing nonglaucomatous optic neuropathies. J Neuroophthalmol. 2007;27(3):176–9. https://doi.org/10.1097/WNO.0b013e31814b1ac4.

56. Mwanza JC, Kim HY, Budenz DL, et al. Residual and dynamic range of retinal nerve fiber layer thickness in glaucoma: comparison of three OCT platforms. Invest Ophthalmol Vis Sci. 2015;56(11):6344–51. https://doi.org/10.1167/iovs.15-17248.

57. Loewen NA, Zhang X, Tan O, et al. Combining measurements from three anatomical areas for glaucoma diagnosis using Fourier-domain optical coherence tomography. Br J Ophthalmol. 2015;99:1224–9. https://doi.org/10.1136/bjophthalmol-2014-305907.

58. Leite MT, Zangwill LM, Weinreb RN, et al. Structure-function relationships using the Cirrus spectral domain optical coherence tomograph and standard automated perimetry. J Glaucoma. 2012;21(1):49–54. https://doi.org/10.1097/IJG.0b013e31822af27a.

59. Garway-Heath DF, Poinoosawmy D, Fitzke FW, Hitchings RA. Mapping the visual field to the optic disc in normal tension glaucoma eyes. Ophthalmology. 2000;107(10):1809–15.

60. Kanamori A, Naka M, Nagai-Kusuhara A, et al. Regional relationship between retinal nerve fiber layer thickness and corresponding visual field sensitivity in glaucomatous eyes. Arch Ophthalmol. 2008;126:1500–6. https://doi.org/10.1001/archopht.126.11.1500.

61. Harwerth RS, Wheat JL, Fredette MJ, Anderson DR. Linking structure and function in glaucoma. Prog Retin Eye Res. 2010;29:249–71. https://doi.org/10.1016/j.preteyeres.2010.02.001.

62. Medeiros FA, Lisboa R, Weinreb RN, et al. A combined index of structure and function for staging glaucomatous damage. Arch Ophthalmol. 2012;130:1107–16. https://doi.org/10.1001/archophthalmol.2012.827.

63. Raza AS, Hood DC. Evaluation of the structure–function relationship in glaucoma using a novel method for estimating the number of retinal ganglion cells in the human retina. Invest Ophthalmol Vis Sci. 2015;56(9):5548–56. https://doi.org/10.1167/iovs.14-16366.

Macular Imaging by Optical Coherence Tomography for Glaucoma

3

Ahnul Ha and Ki Ho Park

Macular Evaluation in Glaucoma

Optic nerve head (ONH) and retinal nerve fiber layer (RNFL) analyses are the standard tools for glaucoma diagnosis and management. Recently, the emergence of spectral-domain optical coherence tomography (SD-OCT) has detoured investigations toward the clinical significance of the detection of glaucomatous ganglion cell damage in the area of the macula. The focus of time-domain optical coherence tomography (TD-OCT) had been on RNFL thickness measurement, because given the comparatively low resolution and poor sampling density of TD-OCT, inner retinal layer segmentation was not reliable [1]. SD-OCT overcame such technical problems in the segmentation of macular layers, and thus, macular imaging protocols became one of the important diagnostic tools of glaucoma detection.

Imaging the macular area by optical coherence tomography (OCT) can provide information regarding the detection of glaucomatous retinal ganglion cell (RGC) damage. Macular thickness can effectively reflect glaucomatous damage, because the macula contains more than half of the RGCs in a multilayered pattern and the RGC body is as much as 20 times larger than the diameter of its axon [2]. The macular area also is notable for its consistency, particularly the fact that it is less affected than the peripapillary RNFL (pRNFL) by interindividual structural variation or non-neural structures such as blood vessels [3, 4].

Principles of Macular Imaging

The low reflectivity of the ganglion cell layer (GCL) is the principal challenge for SD-OCT segmentation algorithms. Given the difficulty of differentiating the GCL and inner plexiform layer (IPL) boundary or the GCL from the RNFL internally, a number of manufacturers have utilized different inner retinal layer combinations in diagnosing glaucoma. Optovue RTVue OCT offers ganglion cell complex (GCC) thickness measurements. The GCC includes the three most inner retinal layers: the RNFL, GCL, and IPL. As such, it contains the ganglion cells' axons, cell bodies, and dendrites, which are preferentially affected by glaucoma. Posterior Pole Asymmetry analysis by Spectralis OCT (Heidelberg Engineering) offers the ability to measure the macula's total retinal thickness, as opposed to segmenting its different layers. Intra-eye asymmetry analysis can be used to compare the inferior and superior

A. Ha · K. H. Park (✉)
Department of Ophthalmology, Seoul National University College of Medicine, Seoul, Korea

Department of Ophthalmology, Seoul National University Hospital, Seoul, Korea
e-mail: kihopark@snu.ac.kr

© Springer Nature Switzerland AG 2020
R. Varma et al. (eds.), *Advances in Ocular Imaging in Glaucoma*, Essentials in Ophthalmology,
https://doi.org/10.1007/978-3-030-43847-0_3

halves of the macula [5]. Additionally, inter-eye asymmetry analysis allows for one-to-one comparison of between-eye differences in superpixel thickness. This method also provides for high sensitivity and specificity [6]. The current version of Spectralis OCT Glaucoma Module Premium Edition can segment individual macular layers but does not provide any statistical analysis capability. Both the SD-OCT and swept-source optical coherence tomography (SS-OCT) systems are available from Topcon Medical Systems. The SS-OCT system, named DRI-OCT Triton, scans the peripapillary area and macula by way of a single 9 × 12 mm scan and can concurrently measure GCC and GCIPL thicknesses.

Cirrus HD-OCT (Carl Zeiss Meditec), with its ganglion cell analysis (GCA) software, provides for analysis of both the ganglion cell layer and inner plexiform layer (GCL + IPL = GCIPL). It identifies the RNFL and IPL outer boundaries and yields GCIPL thickness as the difference between them. This principle is based on the fact that excluding the RNFL from inner retinal thickness measurements can decrease variability [3]. Cirrus HD-OCT has, for the macular cube, two scan options: the default one, which is a 512 × 128 grid consisting of 128 horizontal B-scans each comprising 512 A-scans, and a 200 × 200 macular scan algorithm offering 200 horizontal B-scans each consisting of 200 A-scans. The 512 × 128 algorithm carries out 65,536 A-scans and allows for higher horizontal resolution relative to the 200 × 200 cube scan, which consists of 40,000 A-scans with higher resolution in the vertical direction. The 200 × 200 macular cube, however, has a shorter acquisition time and can be useful for patients who have less-than-optimal fixation. As such, Cirrus HD-OCT can provide macular GCIPL thickness according to the elliptical shape, specifically within the annulus of the inner vertical and horizontal diameters of 1.0 mm and 1.2 mm and the outer vertical and horizontal diameters of 4.0 mm and 4.8 mm, respectively.

A macular GCA report provides the following: (1) the average, minimum, and six-sector (superotemporal, superior, superonasal, inferonasal, inferior, and inferotemporal) GCIPL thickness parameters, (2) a GCIPL thickness map, and (3) a GCIPL deviation map. These thickness parameters also present color codes (i.e., green, normal range; yellow, outside 95% percent normal limit; red, outside 99 percent normal limit) for comparison with the internal normative database. The GCIPL thickness map offers a color-coded display of GCIPL thicknesses with a reference color bar. The GCIPL deviation map represents the deviation from the internal normative database; it indicates yellow or red to represent GCIPL thickness that is less than the lower 5% or 1% of normative data, respectively, as well as uncolored areas within the normal limits. Diagnostic classification by means of color coding provides intuitive results, thereby enabling clinicians to judge the presence and characteristics of macular damage effectively in an at-a-glance view.

Interpretation of Macular OCT

Cirrus HD-OCT's Macular Report (Fig. 3.1)

1. *Patient Data and Signal Strength*: The patient's name and date of birth (DOB) are checked for comparison with the normative database's age-matched data. Note that DOB errors can significantly affect results. The scan's quality control metric is signal strength, and it is recommended by the manufacturer to repeat scans of signal strength less than six.
2. *Thickness Map*: Because Cirrus HD-OCT measures GCL and IPL together, the thickness map provides GCIPL thickness measurements in a cube of 6 × 6 mm, focusing on an elliptical annulus centered on the fovea. The automatic fovea-finder program determines the location of the fovea. The interpreter, however, has to first confirm that placement is correct. The thickness measurements and color codes are not related to the normative database's values, i.e., they are the raw GCIPL thickness data on the macula as scanned. Cool

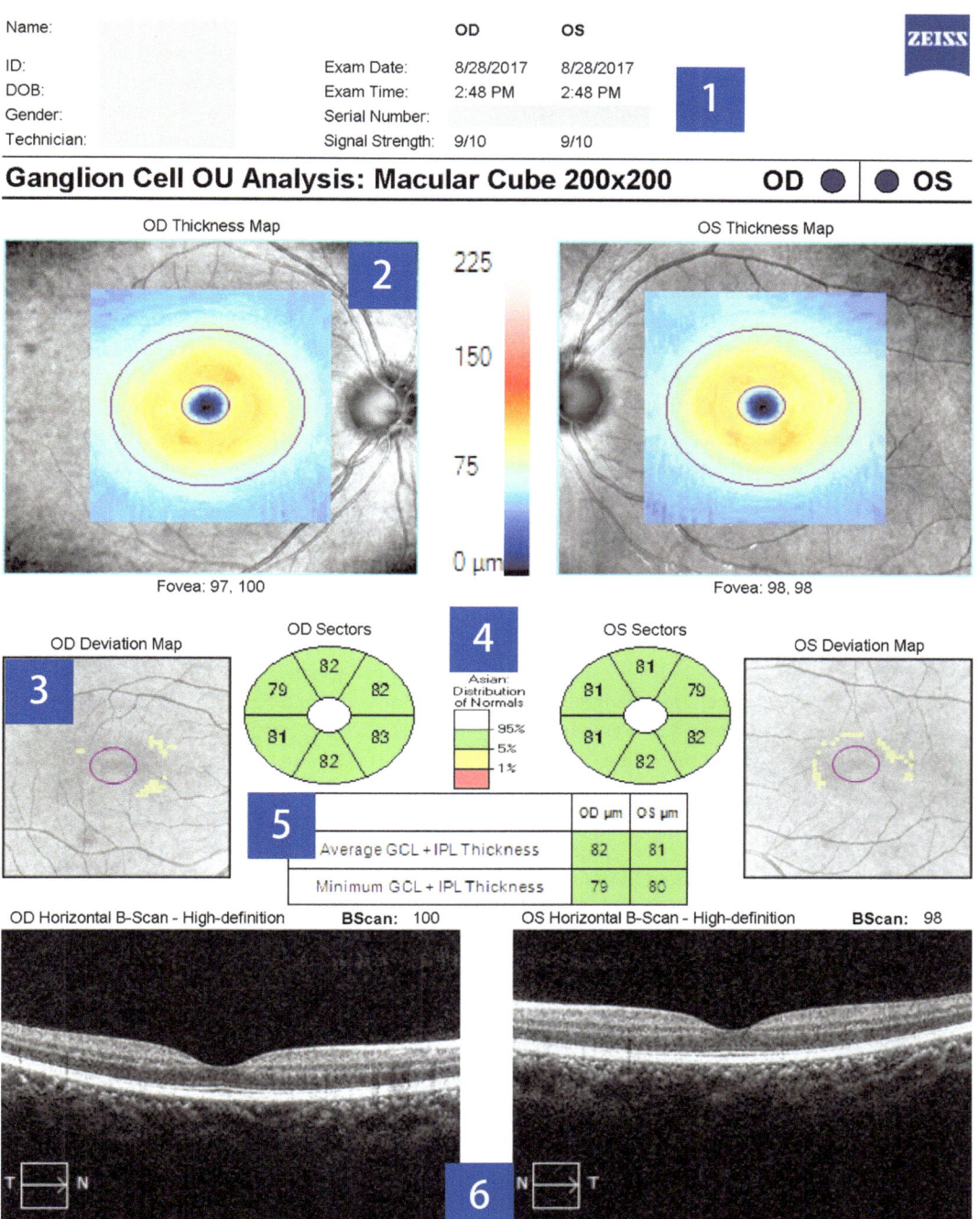

Fig. 3.1 Cirrus HD-OCT's Ganglion Cell OU analysis (based on macular cube's 200 × 200 printout). The printout's sections are explained in the subsection 1.3.1 (the blue squares' label numbers correspond to the heading numbers used therein)

colors (blue, green) are employed to represent thinner GCIPL, while warm colors (yellow, red) represent thicker GCIPL.

3. *Deviation Map*: The GCIPL thicknesses as measured across the 6 × 6 mm cube are compared with the normative database's age-matched data and overlaid on the macula's infrared en face image. The approach used for calculation of GCIPL thicknesses at superpixels is similar to those utilized for the RNFL deviation map of the Optic Disc Cube's RNFL and ONH OU analysis. The device measures GCIPL thicknesses throughout the 6 × 6 mm data cube, each A-scan translating into a 30 μm-square pixel. It combines 16 adjacent pixels to create superpixels of 16 A-scans (4 × 4 pixel squares). Each superpixel covers an approximately 120 × 120 μm area. These are then compared with the data of the normative database; no overlay color code is used to represent areas of normal thickness. Superpixels with GCIPL thicknesses between the first and fifth percentiles of prediction limit for normal subjects are flagged in yellow. Superpixels having a GCIPL value thinner than the first percentile cutoff point for normal subjects are displayed in red on the en-face OCT image. In summary, any region not coded red or yellow can be considered to be within or above the normal limits.

4. *The Sector Map*: The 4.8 × 4.0 mm oval region centered on the fovea consists of a central 1.2 × 1.0 mm diameter elliptical region that represents the fovea where GCIPL thickness is minimal as well as an outer elliptical region for which sectorial measurements are provided. This elliptical annulus is divided into three equal-size pie-shape sectors in the superior and inferior regions. Measurements beyond the normative database's range are shaded in gray. Measurements that fall within the normal measurements' thickest 5% are displayed in white; those within the 5–95% prediction limits are shown in green (normal); thickness measurements falling between 1% and 5% of the normative database's prediction limits are considered borderline abnormal

and, as such, are marked in yellow. Finally, measurements displayed in red are considered to be outside the normal limits and to have thickness values below the normative database measurements' thinnest 1%.

5. *Thickness Table*: The thickness table displays the average and minimum GCIPL thickness measurements in the elliptical annulus. The color codes are the same as for the sector map.

6. *Horizontal Tomogram of the Macula*: This tomogram (B-scan) serves the following purposes. Initially, the interpreter confirms the tomogram passes through the fovea. If so, it is assumed that the elliptical annulus was positioned correctly by the automatic fovea finder and the aforementioned maps provided data are reliable. Second, macular pathologies that might affect the analysis can be detected.

Cirrus HD-OCT PanoMap Analysis

The PanoMap analysis combines the 512 × 128 Macular Cube or 200 × 200 Macular Cube with the 200 × 200 Optic Disc Cube scan into a single report. This integration of a wide-field view of the RNFL and ONH analysis with Ganglion Cell OU and Macular Thickness analysis provides the interpreter the opportunity to evaluate the macula, peripapillary area, and disc altogether (Fig. 3.2). The color codes and principles of PanoMap report interpretation are similar to those of the RNFL/ONH and GCA reports.

Spectralis OCT Posterior Pole Asymmetry Analysis (Fig. 3.3)

1. *Patient and Test Information*: Displays general patient information in the form of patient name, ID, diagnosis, DOB, examination date, and gender.

2. *Posterior Pole Thickness Map*: In each 3° × 3° superpixel on the 8 × 8 grid, the average retinal thickness is displayed. The warmer (more red) the color on the map indicates, the thicker

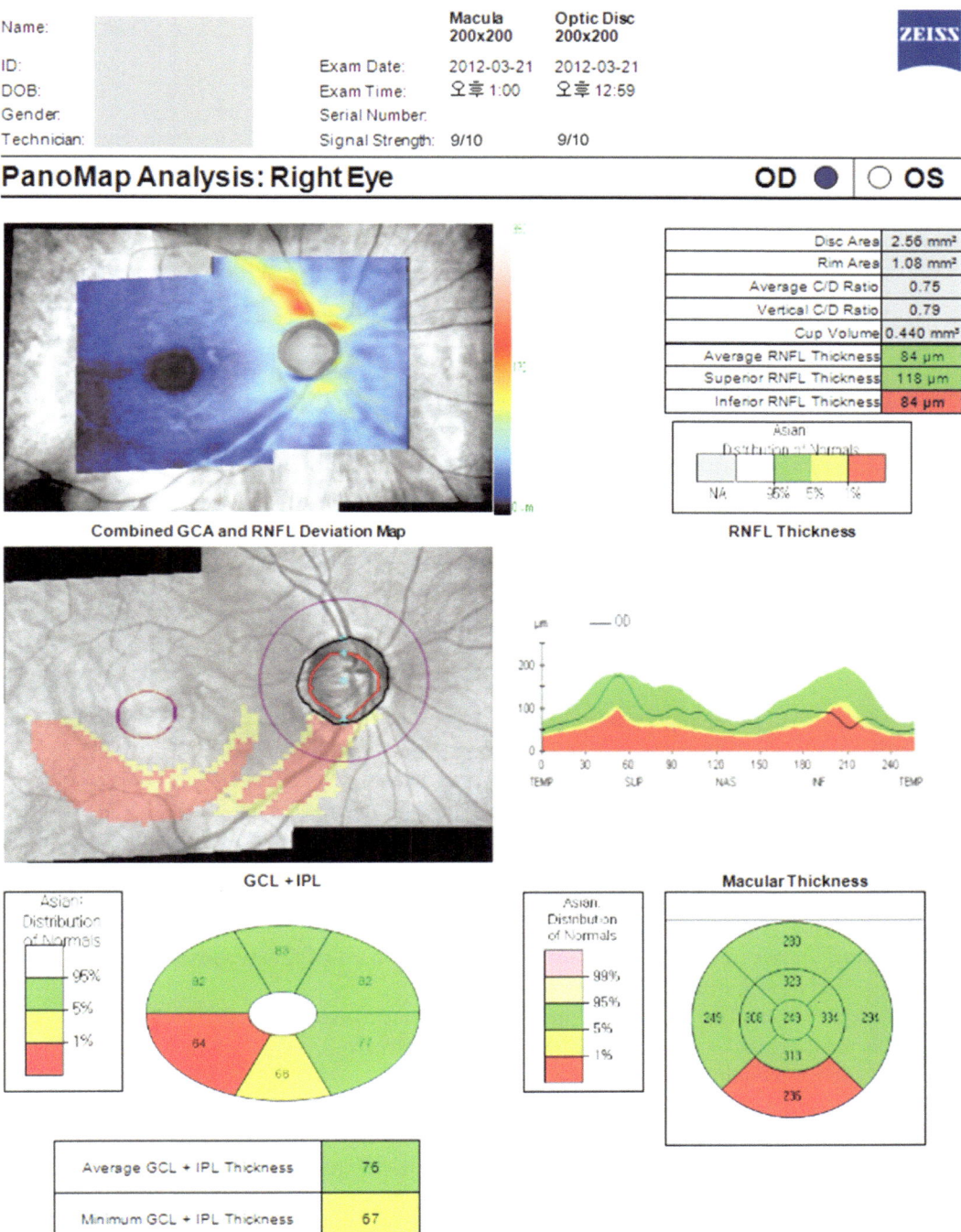

Fig. 3.2 PanoMap analysis is a combination of the 200×200 Optic Disc Cube and 200×200 Macular Cube scans. A peripapillary retinal nerve fiber layer TSNIT plot and a macular full thickness map are additionally included

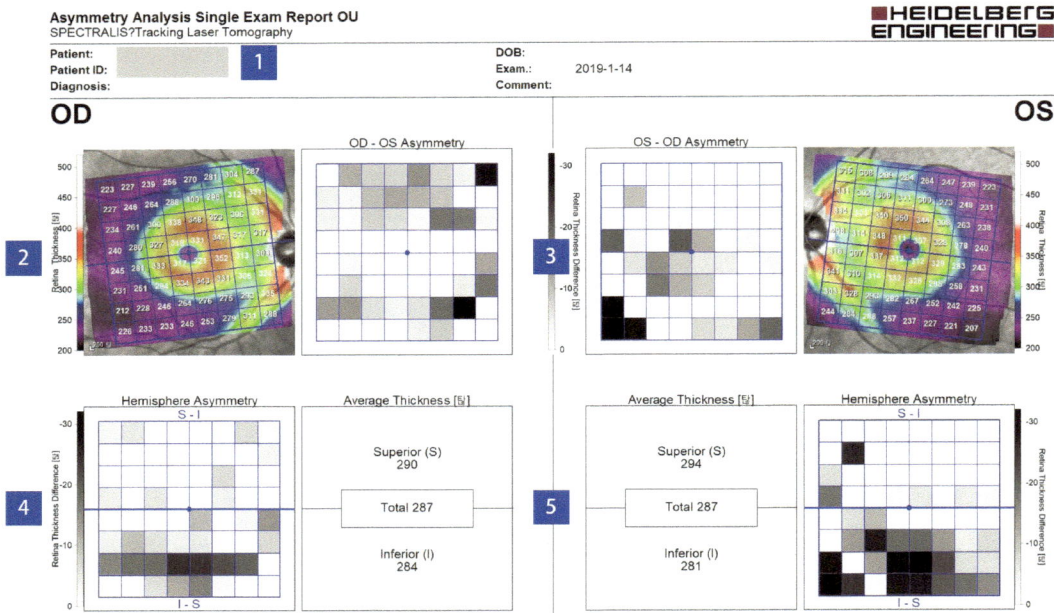

Fig. 3.3 Bilateral posterior-pole asymmetry analysis of subject without glaucoma. Parts of the printout are explained in the subsection 1.3.3 (the blue squares' label numbers correspond to the heading numbers used therein)

the retinal area. The compressed color scale on the map's right side is utilized to localize the smallest retinal thickness differences between adjacent areas.

3. *Interocular Asymmetry Map*: The retinal thicknesses at 64 superpixels in one eye are compared with the corresponding measurements in the other eye. Superpixels with gray shades represent reduced thicknesses relative to corresponding superpixels in the other eye. The gray scale intensity reflects the magnitudes of difference between the eyes' corresponding superpixels.

4. *Hemisphere Asymmetry Map*: The average retinal thickness in superpixels in one hemisphere is compared with the corresponding value in the opposite hemisphere. Superpixels showing any shades of gray in one hemisphere indicate reduced thicknesses relative to those in the corresponding hemisphere. The intensity of the gray color is a function of the degree of difference between the two hemi-

spheres' corresponding superpixels (black: ≥30 μm difference).

5. *Average Thickness Chart*: The averaged retinal thickness of the central 24° × 24° area is provided along with superior and inferior hemisphere thickness measurements.

Diagnosis of Glaucoma

Glaucomatous Change on Macular GCA Map

On the macular GCA deviation map, glaucomatous damage is represented as follows (Fig. 3.4): yellow-colored and red-colored areas indicative of decreased macular GCIPL thickness presented in arcuate to crescent shape, located predominantly in temporal macular regions along the horizontal raphe and usually located also within the same hemifield as corresponding RNFL defect and optic disc neuroretinal rim loss.

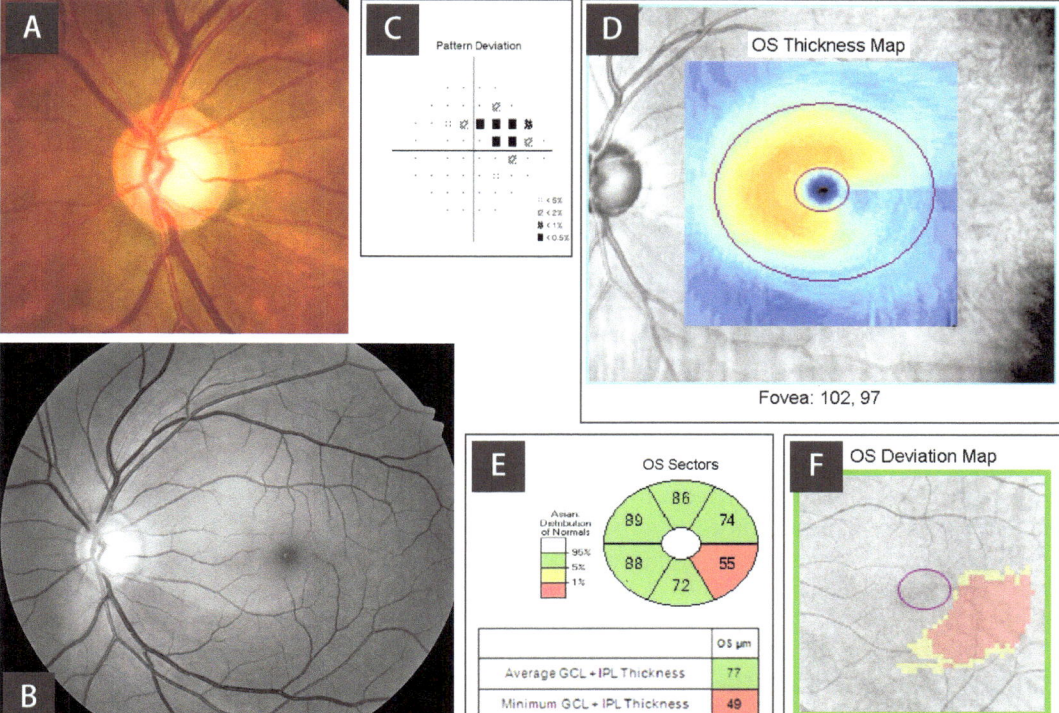

Fig. 3.4 Images of left eye diagnosed with open-angle glaucoma. (**A, B**) Note the inferior neuroretinal rim thinning and inferotemporal retinal nerve fiber layer (RNFL) defect with (**C**) corresponding superior visual field defect. Corresponding (**D–F**) macular ganglion cell–inner plexi-form layer (GCIPL) defect is demonstrated on optical coherence tomography (OCT). The glaucomatous macular GCIPL defect in the macular ganglion cell analysis demonstrates a typical arcuate shape that apparently was related to the peripapillary RNFL defect

Diagnostic Ability in Early Glaucoma

Disease severity affects the glaucoma-diagnostic ability of SD-OCT; therefore, investigators have been keen to validate the diagnostic performance of macular parameters for early disease stages. According to the obtained results, macular parameters have shown excellent, RNFL-comparable diagnostic ability in glaucoma-suspect and preperimetric glaucoma patients [7–11]. The macular parameter demonstrating the best diagnostic performance was inferotemporal GCIPL thickness; there was no significant difference between the best pRNFL (7 o'clock sector) and ONH (rim area) parameters in detection of preperimetric glaucoma [12]. Moreover, for preperimetric glaucoma, the macular GCIPL deviation map has shown diagnostic performance comparable to the pRNFL deviation map

[13]. Relevantly, too, good early-glaucoma detection ability (−6 dB <visual field mean deviation) has been demonstrated for macular GCA maps, the rate of detection ranging from 79.4% (thickness map) to 87.8% (deviation map) [8].

Diagnostic Ability in Myopic Eyes

Detection of glaucomatous damage in patients with high degrees of myopia is often challenging due to unique ocular characteristics including tilted optic disc and peripapillary atrophy. It has been reported that macular inner retinal thickness, relative to pRNFL thickness, is less affected by myopia degree or myopic-change-related ONH morphology [4, 13]. And, as expected, macular parameters have demonstrated comparable-to-pRNFL diagnostic performance, even in myopic eyes [14–16]. The best parameters for discrimination of normal from glaucomatous eyes in a highly myopic group were deemed to be inferior RNFL (AUROC 0.900) and inferotemporal GCIPL thickness (AUROC 0.852) [15]. Inferotemporal macular GCIPL thickness, in fact, has been found to be best for glaucoma detection in cases of myopic preperimetric glaucoma as well [16]. Moreover, in diagnostic ability, it was found to be significantly better than average or inferior RNFL thickness and rim area. Thus far, the majority of relevant studies agree that macular parameters provide—even for highly myopic eyes—reliable diagnostic parameters. However, for accurate interpretation of glaucomatous change in such cases, due consideration must be given to segmentation error, artifacts, or possible instances of false-positive innate abnormality relative to the internal normative database.

Clinical Tips for Use of Macular GCA Maps in Cases of Diagnostic Uncertainty

Other than GCIPL thickness measurements, the chief advantages of macular GCA are the thickness and deviation maps showing GCIPL defect. The characteristics of GCIPL defect can aid clinicians' differentiation of glaucoma from other macular diseases or optic neuropathies. Interestingly, based on detection of superior–inferior GCIPL thickness difference across the temporal horizontal raphe (i.e., the GCIPL hemifield test), Kim and colleagues were able to offer a practical tip on how to use the GCIPL thickness map: such positivity of hemifield difference suggests a strong probability of glaucomatous damage [17]. This can be useful for discrimination of early structural damage, especially in highly myopic patients with depigmented fundus and RNFL defect that is not visible or in patients with preperimetric or early perimetric glaucoma [18]. In addition, detection of superior–inferior GCIPL thickness difference across the temporal horizontal raphe can be an effective tool for discrimination of glaucomatous from non-glaucomatous GCIPL thinning. A steplike configuration near the temporal raphe (the so-called positive temporal raphe sign, Fig. 3.5) appears on OCT macular thickness maps along with absence of relative afferent pupillary defect can be regarded as glaucomatous GCIPL thinning [19].

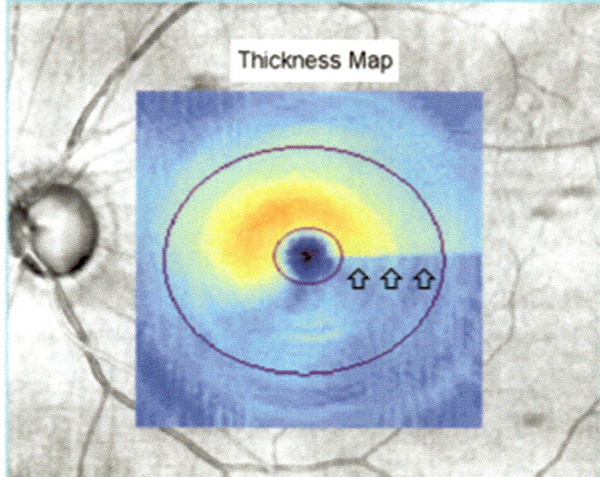
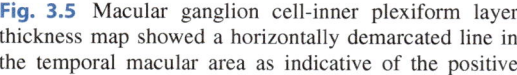
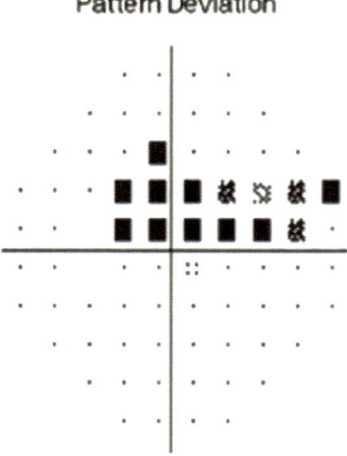

Fig. 3.5 Macular ganglion cell-inner plexiform layer thickness map showed a horizontally demarcated line in the temporal macular area as indicative of the positive temporal raphe sign (arrows). Definite functional glaucomatous defect shown in corresponding visual field (i.e., superior hemifield)

Detection of Glaucoma Progression

A longitudinal study of glaucomatous and healthy eyes reported that GCIPL, as compared with pRNFL, showed similar sensitivity levels for detection of glaucoma progression [20]. RNFL evaluation is less sensitive than the visual field for tracking of advanced cases of progression; this is due to a floor effect, which occurs once the residual RGC layer has nearly diminished [21, 22]. A longitudinal study of visual-field-determined advanced glaucoma eyes demonstrated the average macular thickness loss rate was significantly higher in the progressed group than in the stable or undetermined groups over a mean follow-up period of 2.2 years. Furthermore, the average pRNFL thickness loss rates among the groups were similar, which suggests macular thickness assessment could be better for detection of progression in cases of advanced glaucoma [23, 24]. However, additional longitudinal studies including longer follow-up durations must be completed.

Progression Analysis Software

OCT manufacturers use various strategies for determination of glaucoma progression. Guided Progression Analysis (GPA) is the software package of the Humphrey Field Analyzer (HFA) (Carl Zeiss Meditec, Inc., Dublin, California). Similar to the HFA's GPA, Cirrus HD-OCT provides both event-based and trend-based analyses for detection of glaucoma progression. Currently, this is the only commercial OCT software package offering both event-based and trend-based analyses for RNFL calculation circle measurements, pRNFL thickness maps, macular ganglion cell thickness maps, and ONH parameters.

Basic Concepts of Cirrus HD-OCT's Ganglion Cell GPA

The ganglion cell GPA of Cirrus HD-OCT tracks changes of macular GCIPL thickness. Typically, GPA's event analysis employs the first two scans as baseline data and then compares as many as six subsequent scans to the baseline images. The user can choose any two available scans as baseline images and can look for progression after a specific date. One of the most important properties of Cirrus HD-OCT GPA is its non-dependence on the normative database. GPA makes all of its comparisons between the mean of the two baseline images and a patient's follow-up scans; as such, the results are not related to any normative database-derived data. This independence prevents any errors related to anatomical variations or refractive errors or to race- or age-related differences. The results can be considered truly specific to the given individual.

Reading Cirrus HD-OCT's Ganglion Cell GPA Report (Fig. 3.6)

1. *Patient Data*: Check the patient's name and date of birth
2. *Baseline and Follow-up Maps*: The initial four rows provide the date, patient ID, registration method, signal strength, and average GCIPL values throughout the elliptical annulus. The second part includes serial maps displaying the actual values measured inside of the macular elliptical annulus using the false color code scheme, as explained previously. As is the case in the RNFL thickness map progression analysis, these are the raw thickness data for a scanned eye, and the color coding is independent of the normative database. Before the results can be evaluated, these maps need to be checked for imaging artifacts. On the maps, gross thickness-value changes can be observed.
3. *Thickness Change Maps (Event Analysis)*: These maps display deviations from the two baseline measurements. If the change of thickness exceeds the test-retest variability for specific superpixels relative to the baselines, those pixels are flagged in orange as "possible loss." In the subsequent scan, if the same superpixels show thinning beyond the test-retest variability, they are flagged in red as "likely loss." Finally, if superpixels display thickening

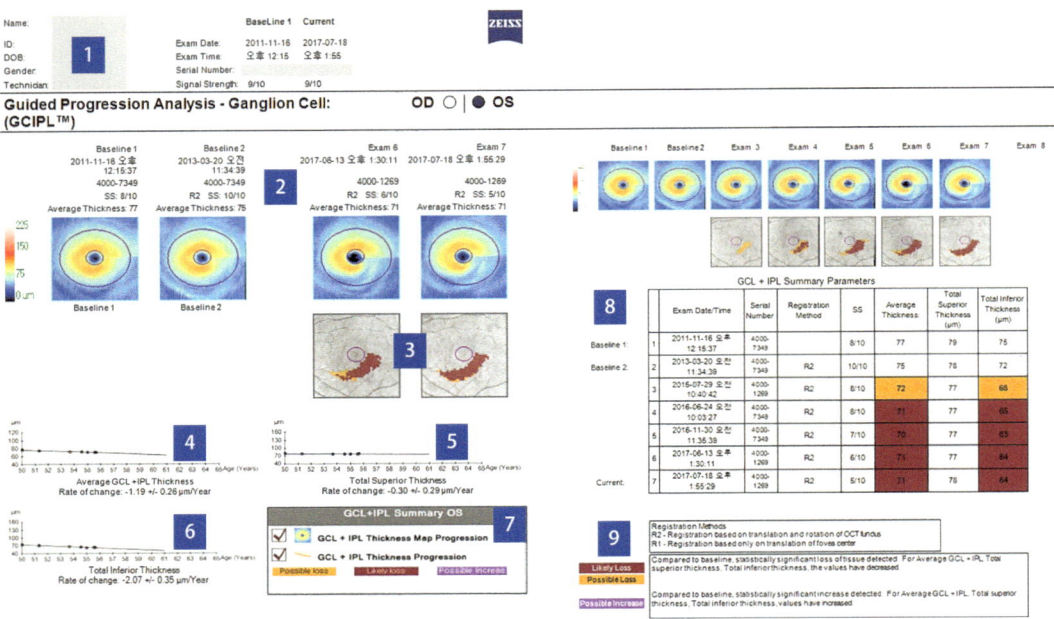

Fig. 3.6 Two-page printout of Cirrus HD-OCT's macular ganglion cell Guided Progression Analysis (GPA) report. Sections of the printout are explained in the subsection 1.5.3 (the blue squares' label numbers correspond to the heading numbers used therein)

beyond the expected test-retest variability, they are flagged in lavender as "possible increase," which can result from macular edema, vitreomacular traction, artifacts or just measurement noise. Changing superpixels are flagged if change is present in 20 or more pixels that are adjacent to each other.

4. *Average Thickness Change Plot (Trend Analysis)*: Average values of elliptical annulus thickness are plotted as a function of time. Each measurement is shown in a small black circle if the change does not exceed the test-retest variability relative to the baseline. If there is thinning beyond the test-retest variability, the circle representing the scan is colored orange; if the following GCL + IPL measurement continues to be significantly thinner than the baseline, the circle is colored red. If both "likely loss" (on event analysis) and a significant linear trend ($p < 0.05$) exist, the rate of loss is estimated by plotting of a linear regression line. The regression line's confidence interval is shaded around it in gray.

The slope of the regression line also is presented as the rate of change in μm/year (± 95% confidence interval). This rate of change is presented only if there are four or more scans spanning 2 years or more.

5. *Total Superior Thickness Change Plot (Trend Analysis)*: Superior-half GCIPL measurements for the elliptical annulus are plotted as a function of time. The same manner of presentation as for the Average Thickness Change Plot (described above) is used here.

6. *Total Inferior Thickness Change Graph (Trend Analysis)*: Inferior-half GCIPL measurements for the elliptical annulus are plotted as a function of time. Again, the same manner of presentation as for Average Thickness Change Plot is used here. In most early stage glaucoma patients, the initial signs of progression are observed in the macula's inferior temporal sector.

7. *Summary*: The two analysis types employed in ganglion cell GPA are the thickness progression map and thickness progression analysis.

Each analysis has a box that is checked in cases where there is significant observable change. An orange check—"possible loss"—indicates that progression is detected on one scan; a red check —"likely loss"— denotes a progression on two, consecutive scans, and a lavender check denotes "possible increase."

8. *Summary Parameters Table*: The table, which is found on the ganglion cell GPA report's page two, summarizes the data utilized to draw the page one plots. An event analysis of the measurements is performed. The cells containing values indicative of change beyond test-retest variability relative to the baseline values are colored orange as "possible loss," meaning progression is detected on one scan; red, as "likely loss" denoting progression detected on two, consecutive scans, and lavender, in cases where "possible increase" in thickness is detected.

9. *Legend*: The legend defines the available image registration modes, the color codes, as well as the criteria for "possible loss," "likely loss," and "possible increase."

Spectralis OCT's Posterior Pole Retinal Thickness Change Report

The report, including the retinal thickness change map, indicates the retina's full-thickness change as measured by the Posterior Pole Horizontal Algorithm. The retinal thickness change map is a color-coded map of posterior pole retinal thickness. The color scale, located on the right side of the map, is used to define even the smallest retinal thickness differences among superpixels for the selected tests, increasing intensities of red representing increased thinning, and green representing thickening. No change is indicated in black. This color scale is completely different from both the false-color code used with the horizontal tomogram and the color code used with the retinal thickness maps. It should be noted that red color on the retina thickness change map denotes thinning, in direct contrast to the retinal thickness maps.

Relationship Between RNFL and Macular Parameters

Many studies have tried to integrate pRNFL with macular GCIPL parameters and to determine the spatial relations between them. Dr. Hood at Columbia University, hypothesized macular area involvement in cases of early glaucomatous damage and further posited that glaucomatous macular damage typically is associated with local RNFL thinning within a narrow disc region they named the macular vulnerability zone [25]. Kim et al. investigated the temporal relationship of inferior macular GCIPL loss to corresponding pRNFL defect on the OCT deviation map. In early glaucoma eyes, GCIPL change was frequently detected before any corresponding pRNFL change, which suggested as a cause superior GCIPL deviation map sensitivity allowing for earlier detection of any abnormality in the macular area [26]. Considering OCT pRNFL analysis alone can overlook macular damage, it is advisable that GCIPL evaluation be included in imaging algorithms for the purposes of serial observation of glaucoma patients and glaucoma suspects.

With regard to glaucoma progression, a prospective study performed by Hou and colleagues including an average follow-up duration of 5.8 years demonstrated that progressive pRNFL and macular GCIPL thinning, as determined by GPA, are mutually predictive. The study also found integrating macular GCIPL with pRNFL measurements facilitates early detection of worsening disease, as progressive pRNFL thinning and macular GCIPL thinning both can be considered to be indicative of visual field progression [27].

The evidence accumulated suggests that ONH, pRNFL, and macular measurements are all complementary, and the use of multiple parameters enhances sensitivity for glaucomatous change detection. However, use of multiple parameters might increase false-positive rates. Therefore, the availability of multiple structural parameters represents both an opportunity and a challenge as to which issue needs to be addressed thoroughly in further studies.

Artifacts and Anatomical Variations in Macular OCT

Clinicians should be aware of limitations related to some OCT devices' restricted macular scanning area. Glaucomatous eyes showing RNFL defect having a long angular distance from the fovea must be examined with caution, as corresponding macular damage might be located outside of the scanning area [8, 12].

Additionally, in GCIPL-diagnostic classifications for normal, healthy populations, false-positive findings have been reported; this would suggest OCT-based diagnostic classifications should be interpreted with special caution, especially in cases of eyes with long axial length, large fovea–disc angle and small optic discs [28]. Young Hoon Hwang reported abnormal patterns on GCIPL deviation maps for cases with diseases including macular degeneration (ring-shaped pattern), epiretinal membrane (irregular color-coded pattern), and compressive optic neuropathy (vertical hemifield abnormality), all of which demand careful GCIPL deviation map interpretation [29].

Compliance with Ethical Requirements Ahnul Ha and Ki Ho Park declare they have no conflict of interest. No human or animal studies were carried out by the authors for this article. Animal studies: no animal studies were carried out by the authors for this article.

References

1. Medeiros FA, Zangwill LM, Bowd C, Vessani RM, Susanna R Jr, Weinreb RN. Evaluation of retinal nerve fiber layer, optic nerve head, and macular thickness measurements for glaucoma detection using optical coherence tomography. Am J Ophthalmol. 2005;139:44–55.
2. Curcio CA, Allen KA. Topography of ganglion cells in human retina. J Comp Neurol. 1990;300:5–25.
3. Mwanza J-C, Oakley JD, Budenz DL, Chang RT, O'Rese JK, Feuer WJ. Macular ganglion cell–inner plexiform layer: automated detection and thickness reproducibility with spectral domain–optical coherence tomography in glaucoma. Invest Ophthalmol Vis Sci. 2011;52(11):8323–9.
4. Jeong JH, Choi YJ, Park KH, Kim DM, Jeoung JW. Macular ganglion cell imaging study: covariate effects on the spectral domain optical coherence tomography for glaucoma diagnosis. PLoS One. 2016;11:e0160448.
5. Asrani S, Rosdahl JA, Allingham RR. Novel software strategy for glaucoma diagnosis: asymmetry analysis of retinal thickness. Arch Ophthalmol. 2011;129:1205–11.
6. Seo JH, Kim T-W, Weinreb RN, Park KH, Kim SH, Kim DM. Detection of localized retinal nerve fiber layer defects with posterior pole asymmetry analysis of spectral domain optical coherence tomography. Invest Ophthalmol Vis Sci. 2012;53:4347–53.
7. Nouri-Mahdavi K, Nowroozizadeh S, Nassiri N, Cirineo N, Knipping S, Giaconi J, et al. Macular ganglion cell/inner plexiform layer measurements by spectral domain optical coherence tomography for detection of early glaucoma and comparison to retinal nerve fiber layer measurements. Am J Ophthalmol. 2013;156:1297–307.e2.
8. Hwang YH, Jeong YC, Kim HK, Sohn YH. Macular ganglion cell analysis for early detection of glaucoma. Ophthalmology. 2014;121:1508–15.
9. Jeoung JW, Choi YJ, Park KH, Kim DM. Macular ganglion cell imaging study: glaucoma diagnostic accuracy of spectral-domain optical coherence tomography. Invest Ophthalmol Vis Sci. 2013;54:4422–9.
10. Mwanza J-C, Durbin MK, Budenz DL, Sayyad FE, Chang RT, Neelakantan A, et al. Glaucoma diagnostic accuracy of ganglion cell–inner plexiform layer thickness: comparison with nerve fiber layer and optic nerve head. Ophthalmology. 2012;119:1151–8.
11. Sung M-S, Yoon J-H, Park S-W. Diagnostic validity of macular ganglion cell-inner plexiform layer thickness deviation map algorithm using cirrus HD-OCT in preperimetric and early glaucoma. J Glaucoma. 2014;23:e144–e51.
12. Kim MJ, Jeoung JW, Park KH, Choi YJ, Kim DM. Topographic profiles of retinal nerve fiber layer defects affect the diagnostic performance of macular scans in preperimetric glaucoma. Invest Ophthalmol Vis Sci. 2014;55:2079–87.
13. Kim MJ, Park KH, Yoo BW, Jeoung JW, Kim HC, Kim DM. Comparison of macular GCIPL and peripapillary RNFL deviation maps for detection of glaucomatous eye with localized RNFL defect. Acta Ophthalmol Scand. 2015;93:e22–e8.
14. Akashi A, Kanamori A, Ueda K, Inoue Y, Yamada Y, Nakamura M. The ability of SD-OCT to differentiate early glaucoma with high myopia from highly myopic controls and non-highly myopic controls. Invest Ophthalmol Vis Sci. 2015;56:6573–80.
15. Choi YJ, Jeoung JW, Park KH, Kim DM. Glaucoma detection ability of ganglion cell-inner plexiform layer thickness by spectral-domain optical coherence tomography in high myopia. Invest Ophthalmol Vis Sci. 2013;54:2296–304.
16. Seol BR, Jeoung JW, Park KH. Glaucoma detection ability of macular ganglion cell-inner plexiform layer thickness in myopic preperimetric glaucoma. Invest Ophthalmol Vis Sci. 2015;56:8306–13.

17. Kim YK, Yoo BW, Kim HC, Park KH. Automated detection of hemifield difference across horizontal raphe on ganglion cell–inner plexiform layer thickness map. Ophthalmology. 2015;122:2252–60.

18. Kim YK, Yoo BW, Jeoung JW, Kim HC, Kim HJ, Park KH. Glaucoma-diagnostic ability of ganglion cell-inner plexiform layer thickness difference across temporal raphe in highly myopic eyes. Invest Ophthalmol Vis Sci. 2016;57:5856–63.

19. Lee J, Kim YK, Ha A, Kim YW, Baek SU, Kim J-S, et al. Temporal raphe sign for discrimination of glaucoma from optic neuropathy in eyes with macular ganglion cell-inner plexiform layer thinning. Ophthalmology. 2019;126(8):1131–9.

20. Na JH, Sung KR, Baek S, Kim YJ, Durbin MK, Lee HJ, et al. Detection of glaucoma progression by assessment of segmented macular thickness data obtained using spectral domain optical coherence tomography. Invest Ophthalmol Vis Sci. 2012;53:3817–26.

21. Leung CK-S, CYL C, Weinreb RN, Qiu K, Liu S, Li H, et al. Evaluation of retinal nerve fiber layer progression in glaucoma: a study on optical coherence tomography guided progression analysis. Invest Ophthalmol Vis Sci. 2010;51:217–22.

22. Wollstein G, Kagemann L, Bilonick RA, Ishikawa H, Folio LS, Gabriele ML, et al. Retinal nerve fibre layer and visual function loss in glaucoma: the tipping point. Br J Ophthalmol. 2012;96:47–52.

23. Sung KR, Sun JH, Na JH, Lee JY, Lee Y. Progression detection capability of macular thickness in advanced glaucomatous eyes. Ophthalmology. 2012;119:308–13.

24. Shin JW, Sung KR, Lee GC, Durbin MK, Cheng D. Ganglion cell–inner plexiform layer change detected by optical coherence tomography indicates progression in advanced glaucoma. Ophthalmology. 2017;124:1466–74.

25. Hood DC. Improving our understanding, and detection, of glaucomatous damage: an approach based upon optical coherence tomography (OCT). Prog Retin Eye Res. 2017;57:46–75.

26. Kim YK, Ha A, Na KI, Kim HJ, Jeoung JW, Park KH. Temporal relation between macular ganglion cell–inner plexiform layer loss and peripapillary retinal nerve fiber layer loss in glaucoma. Ophthalmology. 2017;124:1056–64.

27. Hou HW, Lin C, Leung CK-S. Integrating macular ganglion cell inner plexiform layer and parapapillary retinal nerve fiber layer measurements to detect glaucoma progression. Ophthalmology. 2018;125:822–31.

28. Kim KE, Jeoung JW, Park KH, Kim DM, Kim SH. Diagnostic classification of macular ganglion cell and retinal nerve fiber layer analysis: differentiation of false-positives from glaucoma. Ophthalmology. 2015;122:502–10.

29. Hwang YH. Patterns of macular ganglion cell abnormalities in various ocular conditions. Invest Ophthalmol Vis Sci. 2014;55:3995–6.

OCTA in Glaucoma

4

Grace M. Richter and Ruikang K. Wang

Optical coherence tomography angiography (OCTA) is a noninvasive, fast, and cost-effective modality that provides high-resolution 3D imaging of the retinal microvasculature [1–3]. OCTA uses the variation in optical coherence tomography (OCT) signal caused by moving particles—namely, red blood cells—as the contrast agent for imaging blood flow. Sequential repeated scans are obtained to extract signals that are indicative of the moving red blood cells, upon which to create the angiographic image of the perfused microvasculature (Fig. 4.1). First FDA approved in 2015, OCTA has significant advantages to its precursor technologies. Fluorescein angiography [4], laser Doppler flowmetry and laser speckle flowgraphy [5–8], Doppler OCT [9, 10], and color Doppler ultrasonography [11, 12] previously demonstrated reduced optic disc perfusion and retrobulbar blood flow in glaucomatous eyes but were limited in their abilities to see the microcirculation. Since 2015, there has been a wealth of literature demonstrating the ability of OCTA to identify glaucoma and even

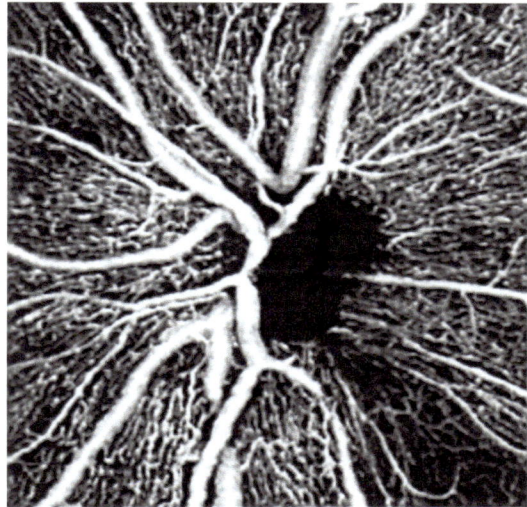

Fig. 4.1 3 × 3 mm OCTA *en face* image of the radial peripapillary capillary layer of a patient's left eye demonstrating an inferotemporal wedge defect from glaucomatous damage

its various stages of severity. These studies have demonstrated its correlations with structural and functional measures of the disease and have suggested potential advantages to traditional OCT assessment of retinal nerve fiber layer thickness. Future longitudinal studies will help to understand the role of OCTA in identifying disease progression and may also aid efforts to understand the role of vascular abnormalities in the pathogenesis of glaucoma. This chapter details

G. M. Richter (✉)
USC Roski Eye Institute, Keck Medicine of University of Southern California, Los Angeles, CA, USA
e-mail: grace.richter@med.usc.edu

R. K. Wang
University of Washington, Department of Bioengineering and Ophthalmology, Seattle, WA, USA

© Springer Nature Switzerland AG 2020
R. Varma et al. (eds.), *Advances in Ocular Imaging in Glaucoma*, Essentials in Ophthalmology,
https://doi.org/10.1007/978-3-030-43847-0_4

evidence for the current utility of OCTA for clinical assessment of glaucoma, highlights its potential as both a clinical and research tool and discusses practical pearls for incorporating it into your practice.

Diagnostic Accuracy of Glaucoma Detection

Optic Disc

In 2012, An et al. and Jia et al. were the first to describe OCTA imaging of the optic disc vasculature in humans [13, 14]. An et al. used the optical microangiography (OMAG)-based algorithm of OCTA and demonstrated the high-resolution relationship between optic disc microvasculature with laminar structure [13]. Jia et al. used the split-spectrum amplitude-decorrelation angiography (SSADA) algorithm and demonstrated reduced ONH perfusion in preperimetric glaucoma eyes compared to normal eyes [14]. Several other studies have since demonstrated significantly reduced microcirculation within the optic nerve head in glaucoma compared to normal eyes [15–20], but area under the receiver operating curve (AUC) measurements of diagnostic accuracy has been relatively low, ranging from 0.57 to 0.82 using various measures of disc perfusion [15, 16, 19]. Utility of optic disc microcirculation measurements for glaucoma diagnosis is limited by segmentation difficulties due to disc anatomy variation and artifacts from large blood vessels, so most recent work has focused on the peripapillary and macular regions.

Peripapillary Area

Significant work has been done on the efficacy of studying the superficial microvasculature in the peripapillary region. Most of these studies have looked specifically at the radial peripapillary capillaries, the microvasculature within the retinal nerve fiber layer. These largely case-control or clinic population studies have demonstrated AUCs for peripapillary vessel density between 0.79 and 0.94 for detection of POAG [16, 21–28]. These studies have varied in terms of OCTA algorithm used, image size used, and minor differences in segmentation algorithms. When analyses for particular segments of the peripapillary region have been done, the inferior and superior quadrants are generally best, as seen with RNFL thickness data [29]. This is supported by understanding that glaucoma damage tends to happen in the inferior and superior regions first [30–32]. It has also been demonstrated that diagnostic accuracy for detection of early glaucoma was greatest for the inferior and superior quadrants; but diagnostic accuracy for detection of moderate to severe glaucoma was good for each quadrant, indicating that early glaucoma damage is typically more focal but advanced disease typically has more diffuse damage [29]. When 4.5×4.5 mm versus 6×6 mm scan sizes have been directly compared with spectral domain OCTA, the 4.5 mm scans outperformed the 6 mm scans, indicating higher digital resolution of the immediate peripapillary area was most important in detecting glaucomatous changes [33].

While most studies focused on measures of perfused vessel density, a few studies have tried to measure the fluid dynamics of the peripapillary microvasculature. Liu et al. reported a peripapillary flow index, which was based on the average decorrelation value and comes from SSADA-based OCTA, and reported an AUC of 0.89 in their small case-control study of 12 normal patients and 12 glaucoma patients. This was slightly lower than their AUC for peripapillary vessel density (VD) of 0.94 [21]. In another case-control study, Chen et al. reported an AUC for flux index, based on the mean flow signal intensity from OMAG-based OCTA of 0.93, which was somewhat higher compared to their AUC for vessel density of 0.82 [25]. In their glaucoma clinic population, Richter et al. reported an AUC for peripapillary flux index of 0.87 compared to their AUC for peripapillary VD of 0.84. In the available studies, flux seemed to outperform VD while flow index appeared to slightly underperform VD measurements. More data is needed to understand the differences between these flow-based parameters and the perfused VD-based parameters for glaucoma.

Macula

There has been mounting interest in the utility of macular OCTA imaging for glaucoma. Inner macular thickness from OCT has previously shown good diagnostic accuracy [34–36], and the macular region has the benefit of avoiding segmentation artifacts from disc and peripapillary anatomic variations such as peripapillary atrophy. Several studies demonstrated reduced superficial macular vessel density in POAG compared to normal, and the superficial microvasculature has been shown to be superior to deeper macular microvasculature [27, 28, 37–46], which makes sense given the superficial location of the ganglion cell bodies and their axons. AUC values have largely ranged from 0.69 to 0.83, with the exception of a case-control study utilizing projection-resolved OCTA reporting an AUC of 0.96. The limitation of case-control studies is that the AUC can be falsely inflated by the use of extremely normal cases rather than the more borderline cases present in a true clinic population. Richter et al. recently conducted an assessment of a true glaucoma clinic population and found an AUC for glaucoma detection of 0.73 for superficial macular VD and 0.76 for superficial macular flux [27]. However, in studies comparing macular VD to GCIPL thickness, structural thickness measurements are still superior to macular VD in terms of diagnostic accuracy [42, 45, 47, 48].

Several studies have begun evaluating the foveal avascular zone (FAZ) in glaucoma using OCTA. While precursor technologies such as fluorescein angiography have previously demonstrated enlarged FAZ in various conditions, the detail of FAZ analysis has improved substantially with OCTA. Kwon et al. reported FAZ size is correlated with VD, ganglion cell–inner plexiform layer (GCIPL) thickness, and central visual field (VF) sensitivity, and FAZ perimeter is a good measure of detecting glaucomatous eyes with central visual field defects compared to those with only peripheral VF defects [38, 39, 49]. Similarly Choi et al. reported those eyes with central visual field defects had lower FAZ circularity than those eyes with peripheral defects [40]. This high-resolution analysis of the FAZ was not possible prior to OCTA and will likely continue to provide additional insight into glaucomatous eyes, particularly those eyes with more central VF defects.

Comparisons Between Anatomic Regions

When considering which anatomic region is best for glaucoma detection, it is useful to look at studies evaluating various regions within the same study population. Using a case-control design and SSADA-based, Rao et al. reported a diagnostic accuracy for VD of 0.73 within the disc, 0.83 in the peripapillary region, and 0.69 in the macula [16]. Using a consecutive glaucoma clinic population and OMAG-based OCTA, Richter et al. reported an AUC of 0.84 for peripapillary VD and 0.73 for macular VD and an AUC of 0.87 for peripapillary flux versus 0.76 for macular flux [27]. Using swept-source OMAG-based OCTA and a case-control design, Trioli et al. reported an AUC of 0.88 for peripapillary VD versus 0.71 for macular VD for detection of glaucoma compared to healthy controls.

They reported an AUC of 0.83 for peripapillary VD versus 0.56 for macular VD for detection of glaucoma compared to glaucoma suspects [50]. Using a case-control design and SSADA-based OCTA, Chen et al. reported a macular VD AUC of 0.94 compared to peripapillary VD of 0.93 [26]. With the exception of Chen's study, these studies reported better diagnostic accuracy for the peripapillary region compared to the macular region. This is similar to the OCT literature which has largely reported the superiority of peripapillary RNFL thickness compared to inner macular thickness measurements for glaucoma detection [51].

Distinguishing Disease Severities

In general, OCTA studies have demonstrated reduced vessel density with increasing glaucoma severity and therefore increasing diagnostic ability with increasing severity of disease [29, 52, 53]. Nonetheless, OCTA is able to distinguish early glaucoma eyes from normal eyes [29, 54], and, in terms of incremental changes between disease stages, these changes seem to be more pronounced at the earlier stages of disease compared to more advanced disease [29, 47]. In a study that included patients with unilateral glaucoma, there was already significant reduction in peripapillary VD in the contralateral "healthy" eye of patients with unilateral glaucoma compared to normal eyes of patients without glaucoma, suggesting that VD and, in fact, the ability to distinguish these non-involved eyes in patients with unilateral POAG from normal eyes, was greater for peripapillary VD than RNFL thickness [55]. These findings are interesting and support the hypothesis that reduced VD may be a marker for sick retinal ganglion cells prior to apoptosis. There is limited data on how OCTA performs at distinguishing between

more advanced stages of glaucoma, although a study by Rao et al. suggested the peripapillary vessel density plateaus beyond a visual field mean deviation of −15 dB, as compared to plateauing around −10 to −15 dB for RNFL thickness, indicating the floor effect for OCTA may be slightly improved compared to RNFL thickness [56]. Additional work is needed to clarify this finding.

Correlation with Structural and Functional Parameters

Overall, there have been strong correlations between perfused VD measurements by OCTA and corresponding structural measures (RNFL thickness or ganglion cell complex thicknesses) and functional measures (visual field) of glaucoma. These correlations have also been demonstrated for focal anatomic areas [25, 28, 29, 50, 57]. The question has been evaluated in several studies whether VD has a stronger correlation with functional versus structural measures, and while more studies [19, 21, 25, 52, 58] than not [24, 29, 52, 53] seem to suggest they correlate with functional measures more, the results overall are inconsistent. One study reported decreased vessel density was significantly associated with severity of visual field damage, independent of structural damage, with the suggestion that reduced vessel density may sometimes be a marker for sick dysfunctional retinal ganglion cells before apoptosis has occurred [58]. If there is truly a stronger correlation of VD with functional measures, this also suggests OCTA parameters are better markers of visual function than structural thickness values and supports the hypothesis that OCTA may be able to detect dysfunctional retinal ganglion cells prior to true apoptosis and loss of tissue. Two studies evaluated glaucomatous eyes with single hemifield defects and reported interesting results with respect to the perimetrically normal hemiretina. The OMAG-based study found reduced OCTA measures with normal RNFL [59], and the second SSADA-based study found both reduced OCTA and OCT measures [55]. These studies suggest there may be early glaucomatous changes detectable with OCTA before structural or functional changes even occur. While the possibility of using OCTA for earlier detection of glaucomatous changes is promising, longitudinal data are needed to clarify these hypotheses.

Progression

Since OCTA has only been FDA approved since 2015, there is limited data on how OCTA performs in detecting glaucomatous progression. Shoji et al. recently reported evidence of macular VD loss over a 14-month follow-up in glaucoma patients with no detectable change in healthy patients [60]. These results suggest OCTA may be able to detect early glaucomatous progression in the macula that may not be evident with currently available glaucoma testing, although these results must be replicated in the future with longer follow-up and should include the peripapillary region as well. If early progression could be reliably detected with OCTA, this would greatly enhance the ability to monitor glaucoma patients and modify treatment in a timely manner to prevent vision loss.

Assessments of Deeper Microvasculature

There has been growing interest in studying the deep peripapillary microvasculature because it may offer insight into the deep optic nerve head microvasculature, which is thought to be subject to vascular insult leading to glaucomatous damage. One limitation in studying the deeper layers in OCTA, particularly spectral-domain, has been that flow projection artifact from the more superficial layers can obscure the deeper microvasculature. Lee et al. were able to demonstrate that peripapillary choroidal microvasculature dropout in glaucoma patients is comparable to that seen with ICG, and thus this is a reliable method to visualize the deeper microvasculature [61]. Recent studies have found deep layer peripapillary microvasculature dropout is more likely in eyes with recent progression [62, 63] and in eyes with, and at the site of, prior disc hemorrhage [63, 64]. Suh et al. reported beta peripapillary atrophy without Bruch's membrane—termed gamma peripapillary atrophy—is associated with deep microvasculature dropout and suggested the exposed scleral flange predisposes to stress and strain on the posterior ciliary arteries [65]. Other factors found to be associated with deep microvasculature dropout include more advanced glaucoma, reduced RNFL VD, thinner choroidal thickness, and lower diastolic blood pressure [66]. These interesting cross-sectional studies provide evidence that this deep dropout is part of glaucomatous damage not previously visualized. Longitudinal studies are needed to understand whether these precede or follow RNFL loss.

Effect of Glaucoma Treatment on Vessel Density

Currently, there is limited data on the effect various glaucoma treatments have on the retinal microcirculation as measured by OCTA. While topical medications may or may not have a vasoactive effect, glaucoma surgical treatments are hypothesized to improve ocular perfusion pressure by reducing intraocular pressure. A sub-analysis in a report by Takusagawa et al. previously suggested topical beta-blocker use may reduce macular vessel density [41]. Chihara et al. compared the effect of topical rho-associated coiled-coil containing protein kinase (ROCK) inhibitor ripasudil versus brimonidine on peripapillary VD and found ripasudil increased peripapillary VD while brimonidine had no effect [67]. Some preliminary work has begun to investigate whether intraocular pressure reduction from trabeculectomy alters vessel density within and around the optic nerve head in glaucoma patients. Shin et al. recently demonstrated over half of eyes had a 30% or more reduction in peripapillary microvascular dropout area 3 months after trabeculectomy, and this was significantly associated with reduction in lamina cribrosa depth. Using swept source OCTA, Kim et al. showed that after trabeculectomy, there was a significant increase in VD at the level of the lamina cribrosa but not in the peripapillary retina. Additional studies are needed to understand the effect topical medications and intraocular pressure reduction in general has on retinal perfusion.

Patient Factors Affecting Vessel Density

While the relationship between microcirculation parameters such as vessel density and glaucoma is becoming more defined, there have been limited studies on other ocular and systemic factors that may also affect retinal microcirculation. A relatively small study of healthy eyes by Rao et al. recently reported hypertension, diabetes, and male gender reduced microcirculation measurements, but age and disc size did not affect microcirculation. An animal study by Jiang et al. demonstrated increased age was in fact associated with reduced retinal capillary filling index under various intraocular pressure challenges due to reduced autoregulation capacity [68]. Data from the African American Eye Disease Study (AFEDS), a large population-based study of more than 1000 healthy eyes, demonstrated advanced age was independently associated with reduced peripapillary microcirculation. AFEDS also reported the independent associations of male gender, longer diabetes duration, longer axial length, and thinner RNFL with reduced peripapillary microcirculation in healthy eyes without preexisting conditions such as glaucoma or diabetic retinopathy [69]. The influence of diabetes on even peripapillary microcirculation emphasizes the impact diabetes is having on capillary beds even when no pathology is otherwise noted. Additionally, this may provide evidence that diabetes may increase risk for glaucoma [70, 71] by affecting the peripapillary or optic nerve microvasculature. The finding associating longer axial length with reduced peripapillary microcirculation in healthy eyes similarly may also provide evidence that myopia increases risk for glaucoma [72] by compromising the peripapillary microvasculature. Longitudinal studies are needed to clarify these hypotheses and whether these factors compromise optic nerve microvasculature. However, the effects of these factors on perfusion need to be considered when clinicians interpret OCTA images.

In these studies as well as others, signal strength has been shown to be an important factor affecting microcirculation measurements and was therefore required to control for during analyses. Signal strength is a measure of the amount of signal reaching the retina and can be degraded by media opacities such as punctate epithelial keratopathy from dry eye, cataract, or vitreous floaters. In fact, it has been shown that even with signal strength ≥7, vessel density measurements are associated with signal strength [73]. This often-overlooked feature will be extremely important to consider not only in future research but also when examining the OCTA data of glaucoma patients longitudinally.

Practical Pearls for Using OCTA in Glaucoma Practice

OCTA imaging is now an add-on capability available on most commercially available spectral-domain OCT devices and images can be easily captured at the same time as routine OCT. In contrast to traditional OCT, where good quality images can usually be captured on the undilated pupil, OCTA images, particularly of the peripapillary region, are of much better quality if performed on the dilated pupil. It is also important for the patient to maintain good positioning without movement during image acquisition, as OCTA images are more sensitive to motion artifact. When following sequential OCTA images of the same patient, it is also important to understand the effect of media opacities such as floaters (Fig. 4.2) or cataract on the signal strength and the resultant vessel density measurements. For example, cataract extraction may result in improved vessel density in patient's eyes.

The qualitative OCTA images of one patient may be extremely helpful in analyzing patients with indeterminate OCT findings. One such example was previously published of a patient with uveitic glaucoma with gliotic changes causing the RNFL thickness to be supranormal but with OCTA demonstrating reduced perfusion in the affected eye [74]. Another example is demonstrated in Fig. 4.3. These images are from a patient whose OCT and VF were indeterminate but whose OCTA image helped to cinch a diagnosis of primary open angle glaucoma.

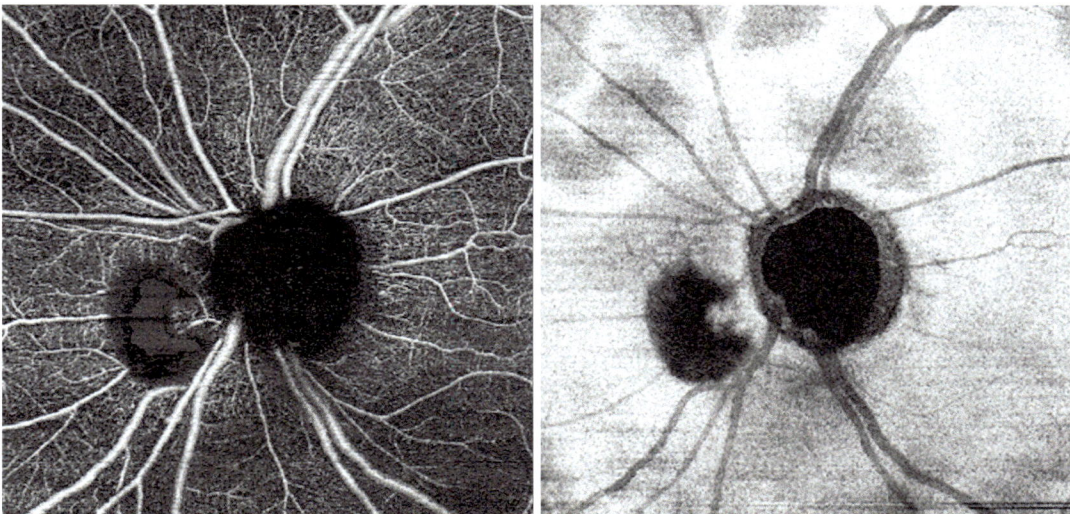

Fig. 4.2 6 × 6 mm OCTA *en face* flow and structural images of a glaucomatous left eye with a large floater causing artifact nasal to the optic disc

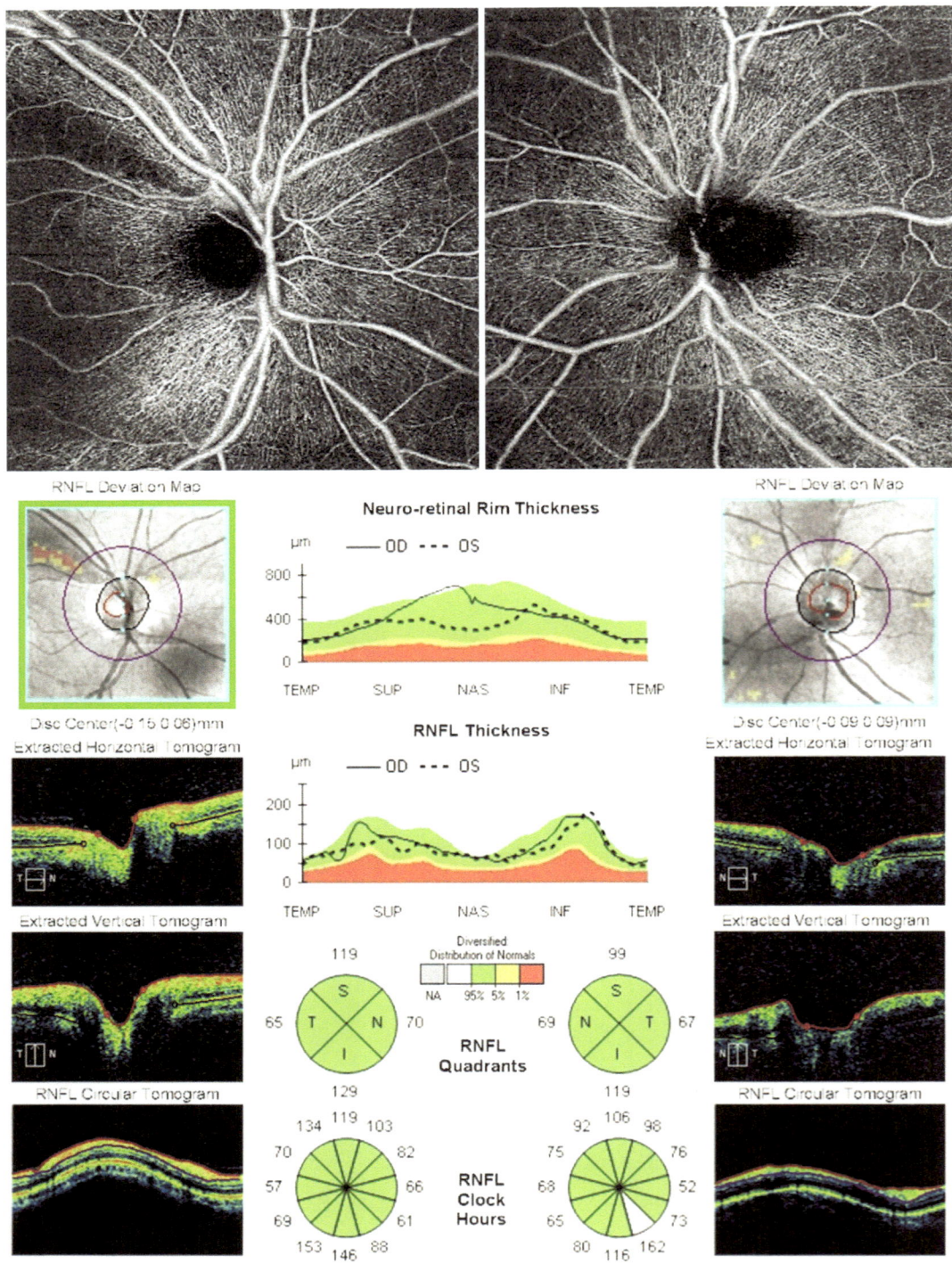

Fig. 4.3 These OCTA and OCT images are of a 72-year-old male who presented for glaucoma suspect evaluation with low-normal intraocular pressures in each eye; visual field was unreliable but showed trace inferior visual field defect in the right eye but normal in the left eye. Optic nerve exam revealed cup-disc ratio of 0.4 in each eye. While RNFL thicknesses were mostly normal, OCTA revealed a classic superotemporal wedge-like defect in the radial peripapillary capillary layer supplying the RNFL of the right eye. The patient was diagnosed with early POAG in the right eye

Conclusion

In summary, significant progress has been made over the last 4 years in how the retinal microcirculation, as measured by OCTA, is affected in glaucoma and how this powerful tool has improved the ability to care for glaucoma patients. OCTA measurements of vessel density are most useful for glaucoma in the immediate peripapillary region within the radial peripapillary capillaries. Nonetheless, meaningful assessments of the deeper optic nerve microvasculature and the superficial macular microcirculation have provided important insights into the vascular pathophysiology of glaucoma. While analyzing OCTA data from patients, it is important to understand the impact of ocular and systemic factors also influencing vessel density. Future longitudinal research will continue to clarify hypotheses related to the vascular mechanisms underlying glaucoma and will help determine whether OCTA can truly detect dysfunctional, but perhaps salvageable, retinal ganglion cells.

Compliance with Ethical Requirements Grace M Richter has received research support in the form of a research device from Zeiss (Dublin, CA). Ruikang K Wang is a consultant, receives research support, and has patents licensed to Zeiss (Dublin, CA). No human studies were carried out by the authors for this article. No animal studies were carried out by the authors for this article.

References

1. Zhang A, Zhang Q, Chen CL, Wang RK. Methods and algorithms for optical coherence tomography-based angiography: a review and comparison. J Biomed Opt. 2015;20(10):100901.
2. Chen CL, Wang RK. Optical coherence tomography based angiography [Invited]. Biomed Opt Express. 2017;8(2):1056–82.
3. Kashani AH, Chen CL, Gahm JK, et al. Optical coherence tomography angiography: a comprehensive review of current methods and clinical applications. Prog Retin Eye Res. 2017;60:66–100.
4. Talusan E, Schwartz B. Specificity of fluorescein angiographic defects of the optic disc in glaucoma. Arch Ophthalmol. 1977;95(12):2166–75.
5. Hamard P, Hamard H, Dufaux J, Quesnot S. Optic nerve head blood flow using a laser Doppler velocimeter and haemorheology in primary open angle glaucoma and normal pressure glaucoma. Br J Ophthalmol. 1994;78(6):449–53.
6. Michelson G, Groh MJ, Langhans M. Perfusion of the juxtapapillary retina and optic nerve head in acute ocular hypertension. Ger J Ophthalmol. 1996;5(6):315–21.
7. Michelson G, Langhans MJ, Groh MJ. Perfusion of the juxtapapillary retina and the neuroretinal rim area in primary open angle glaucoma. J Glaucoma. 1996;5(2):91–8.
8. Yokoyama Y, Aizawa N, Chiba N, et al. Significant correlations between optic nerve head microcirculation and visual field defects and nerve fiber layer loss in glaucoma patients with myopic glaucomatous disk. Clin Ophthalmol. 2011;5:1721–7.
9. Emre M, Orgul S, Gugleta K, Flammer J. Ocular blood flow alteration in glaucoma is related to systemic vascular dysregulation. Br J Ophthalmol. 2004;88(5):662–6.
10. Chung HS, Harris A, Kagemann L, Martin B. Peripapillary retinal blood flow in normal tension glaucoma. Br J Ophthalmol. 1999;83(4):466–9.
11. Meng N, Zhang P, Huang H, et al. Color Doppler imaging analysis of retrobulbar blood flow velocities in primary open-angle glaucomatous eyes: a meta-analysis. PLoS One. 2013;8(5):e62723.
12. Siesky B, Harris A, Racette L, et al. Differences in ocular blood flow in glaucoma between patients of African and European descent. J Glaucoma. 2015;24(2):117–21.
13. An L, Johnstone M, Wang RK. Optical microangiography provides correlation between microstructure and microvasculature of optic nerve head in human subjects. J Biomed Opt. 2012;17(11):116018.
14. Jia Y, Morrison JC, Tokayer J, et al. Quantitative OCT angiography of optic nerve head blood flow. Biomed Opt Express. 2012;3(12):3127–37.
15. Chihara E, Dimitrova G, Amano H, Chihara T. Discriminatory power of superficial vessel density and prelaminar vascular flow index in eyes with glaucoma and ocular hypertension and normal eyes. Invest Ophthalmol Vis Sci. 2017;58(1):690–7.
16. Rao HL, Pradhan ZS, Weinreb RN, et al. Regional comparisons of optical coherence tomography angiography vessel density in primary open-angle glaucoma. Am J Ophthalmol. 2016;171:75–83.
17. Leveque PM, Zeboulon P, Brasnu E, et al. Optic disc vascularization in glaucoma: value of spectral-domain optical coherence tomography angiography. J Ophthalmol. 2016;2016:6956717.
18. Akagi T, Zangwill LM, Shoji T, et al. Optic disc microvasculature dropout in primary open-angle glaucoma measured with optical coherence tomography angiography. PLoS One. 2018;13(8): e0201729.
19. Jia Y, Wei E, Wang X, et al. Optical coherence tomography angiography of optic disc perfusion in glaucoma. Ophthalmology. 2014;121(7):1322–32.
20. Yoshikawa M, Akagi T, Uji A, et al. Pilot study assessing the structural changes in posttrabecular aqueous humor outflow pathway after trabecular meshwork surgery using swept-source optical coherence tomography. PLoS One. 2018;13(6):e0199739.

21. Liu L, Jia Y, Takusagawa HL, et al. Optical coherence tomography angiography of the peripapillary retina in glaucoma. JAMA Ophthalmol. 2015;133(9):1045–52.

22. Yarmohammadi A, Zangwill LM, Diniz-Filho A, et al. Optical coherence tomography angiography vessel density in healthy, glaucoma suspect, and glaucoma eyes. Invest Ophthalmol Vis Sci. 2016;57(9):OCT451–9.

23. Rao HL, Kadambi SV, Weinreb RN, et al. Diagnostic ability of peripapillary vessel density measurements of optical coherence tomography angiography in primary open-angle and angle-closure glaucoma. Br J Ophthalmol. 2017;101(8):1066–70.

24. Geyman LS, Garg RA, Suwan Y, et al. Peripapillary perfused capillary density in primary open-angle glaucoma across disease stage: an optical coherence tomography angiography study. Br J Ophthalmol. 2017;101(9):1261–8.

25. Chen CL, Zhang A, Bojikian KD, et al. Peripapillary retinal nerve fiber layer vascular microcirculation in glaucoma using optical coherence tomography-based microangiography. Invest Ophthalmol Vis Sci. 2016;57(9):OCT475–85.

26. Chen HS, Liu CH, Wu WC, et al. Optical coherence tomography angiography of the superficial microvasculature in the macular and peripapillary areas in glaucomatous and healthy eyes. Invest Ophthalmol Vis Sci. 2017;58(9):3637–45.

27. Richter GM, Chang R, Situ B, et al. Diagnostic performance of macular versus peripapillary vessel parameters by optical coherence tomography angiography for glaucoma. Transl Vis Sci Technol. 2018;7(6):21.

28. Richter GM, Madi I, Chu Z, et al. Structural and functional associations of macular microcirculation in the ganglion cell-inner plexiform layer in glaucoma using optical coherence tomography angiography. J Glaucoma. 2018;27(3):281–90.

29. Richter GM, Sylvester B, Chu Z, et al. Peripapillary microvasculature in the retinal nerve fiber layer in glaucoma by optical coherence tomography angiography: focal structural and functional correlations and diagnostic performance. Clin Ophthalmol. 2018;12:2285–96.

30. Khoueir Z, Jassim F, Poon LY, et al. Diagnostic capability of peripapillary three-dimensional retinal nerve fiber layer volume for glaucoma using optical coherence tomography volume scans. Am J Ophthalmol. 2017;182:180–93.

31. Shin JW, Uhm KB, Lee WJ, Kim YJ. Diagnostic ability of retinal nerve fiber layer maps to detect localized retinal nerve fiber layer defects. Eye (Lond). 2013;27(9):1022–31.

32. Leung CK, Lam S, Weinreb RN, et al. Retinal nerve fiber layer imaging with spectral-domain optical coherence tomography: analysis of the retinal nerve fiber layer map for glaucoma detection. Ophthalmology. 2010;117(9):1684–91.

33. Chang R, Chu Z, Burkemper B, et al. Effect of scan size on glaucoma diagnostic performance using OCT angiography en face images of the radial peripapillary capillaries. J Glaucoma. 2019;28:465.

34. Jeoung JW, Choi YJ, Park KH, Kim DM. Macular ganglion cell imaging study: glaucoma diagnostic accuracy of spectral-domain optical coherence tomography. Invest Ophthalmol Vis Sci. 2013;54(7):4422–9.

35. Mwanza JC, Durbin MK, Budenz DL, et al. Glaucoma diagnostic accuracy of ganglion cell-inner plexiform layer thickness: comparison with nerve fiber layer and optic nerve head. Ophthalmology. 2012;119(6):1151–8.

36. Kim YK, Yoo BW, Jeoung JW, et al. Glaucoma-diagnostic ability of ganglion cell-inner plexiform layer thickness difference across temporal raphe in highly myopic eyes. Invest Ophthalmol Vis Sci. 2016;57(14):5856–63.

37. Akil H, Chopra V, Al-Sheikh M, et al. Swept-source OCT angiography imaging of the macular capillary network in glaucoma. Br J Ophthalmol. 2017:bjophthalmol-2016-309816.

38. Kwon J, Choi J, Shin JW, et al. An optical coherence tomography angiography study of the relationship between foveal avascular zone size and retinal vessel density. Invest Ophthalmol Vis Sci. 2018;59(10):4143–53.

39. Kwon J, Choi J, Shin JW, et al. Glaucoma diagnostic capabilities of foveal avascular zone parameters using optical coherence tomography angiography according to visual field defect location. J Glaucoma. 2017;26(12):1120–9.

40. Choi J, Kwon J, Shin JW, et al. Quantitative optical coherence tomography angiography of macular vascular structure and foveal avascular zone in glaucoma. PLoS One. 2017;12(9):e0184948.

41. Takusagawa HL, Liu L, Ma KN, et al. Projection-resolved optical coherence tomography angiography of macular retinal circulation in glaucoma. Ophthalmology. 2017;124(11):1589–99.

42. Penteado RC, Zangwill LM, Daga FB, et al. Optical coherence tomography angiography macular vascular density measurements and the central 10-2 visual field in glaucoma. J Glaucoma. 2018;27(6):481–9.

43. Lommatzsch C, Rothaus K, Koch JM, et al. OCTA vessel density changes in the macular zone in glaucomatous eyes. Graefes Arch Clin Exp Ophthalmol. 2018;256(8):1499–508.

44. Wu J, Sebastian RT, Chu CJ, et al. Reduced macular vessel density and capillary perfusion in glaucoma detected using OCT angiography. Curr Eye Res. 2018;44(5):533–40.

45. Wan KH, Lam AKN, Leung CK. Optical coherence tomography angiography compared with optical coherence tomography macular measurements for detection of glaucoma. JAMA Ophthalmol. 2018;136(8):866–74.

46. Kromer R, Glusa P, Framme C, et al. Optical coherence tomography angiography analysis of macular flow density in glaucoma. Acta Ophthalmol. 2019;97(2):e199–206.

47. Hou H, Moghimi S, Zangwill LM, et al. Macula vessel density and thickness in early primary open angle glaucoma. Am J Ophthalmol. 2019;199:120–32.

48. Ghahari E, Bowd C, Zangwill LM, et al. Macular vessel density in glaucomatous eyes with focal lmina cribrosa defects. J Glaucoma. 2018;27(4):342–9.
49. Kwon J, Choi J, Shin JW, et al. Alterations of the foveal avascular zone measured by optical coherence tomography angiography in glaucoma patients with central visual field defects. Invest Ophthalmol Vis Sci. 2017;58(3):1637–45.
50. Triolo G, Rabiolo A, Shemonski ND, et al. Optical coherence tomography angiography macular and peripapillary vessel perfusion density in healthy subjects, glaucoma suspects, and glaucoma patients. Invest Ophthalmol Vis Sci. 2017;58(13):5713–22.
51. Oddone F, Lucenteforte E, Michelessi M, et al. Macular versus retinal nerve fiber layer parameters for diagnosing manifest glaucoma: a systematic review of diagnostic accuracy studies. Ophthalmology. 2016;123(5):939–49.
52. Wang X, Jiang C, Ko T, et al. Correlation between optic disc perfusion and glaucomatous severity in patients with open-angle glaucoma: an optical coherence tomography angiography study. Graefes Arch Clin Exp Ophthalmol. 2015;253(9):1557–64.
53. Kumar RS, Anegondi N, Chandapura RS, et al. Discriminant function of optical coherence tomography angiography to determine disease severity in glaucoma. Invest Ophthalmol Vis Sci. 2016;57(14):6079–88.
54. Mansoori T, Sivaswamy J, Gamalapati JS, Balakrishna N. Radial peripapillary capillary density measurement using optical coherence tomography angiography in early glaucoma. J Glaucoma. 2017;26(5):438–43.
55. Yarmohammadi A, Zangwill LM, Diniz-Filho A, et al. Peripapillary and macular vessel density in patients with glaucoma and single-hemifield visual field defect. Ophthalmology. 2017;124(5):709–19.
56. Rao HL, Pradhan ZS, Weinreb RN, et al. Relationship of optic nerve structure and function to peripapillary vessel density measurements of optical coherence tomography angiography in glaucoma. J Glaucoma. 2017;26(6):548–54.
57. Van Melkebeke L, Barbosa-Breda J, Huygens M, Stalmans I. Optical coherence tomography angiography in glaucoma: a review. Ophthalmic Res. 2018;60(3):139–51.
58. Yarmohammadi A, Zangwill LM, Diniz-Filho A, et al. Relationship between optical coherence tomography angiography vessel density and severity of visual field loss in glaucoma. Ophthalmology. 2016;123(12):2498–508.
59. Chen CL, Bojikian KD, Wen JC, et al. Peripapillary retinal nerve fiber layer vascular microcirculation in eyes with glaucoma and single-hemifield visual field loss. JAMA Ophthalmol. 2017;135(5):461–8.
60. Shoji T, Zangwill LM, Akagi T, et al. Progressive macula vessel density loss in primary open-angle glaucoma: a longitudinal study. Am J Ophthalmol. 2017;182:107–17.
61. Lee EJ, Lee KM, Lee SH, Kim TW. Parapapillary choroidal microvasculature dropout in glaucoma: a comparison between optical coherence tomography angiography and indocyanine green angiography. Ophthalmology. 2017;124(8):1209–17.
62. Kwon JM, Suh MH, Weinreb RN, Zangwill LM. Parapapillary deep-layer microvasculature dropout and visual field progression in glaucoma. Am J Ophthalmol. 2019;200:65–75.
63. Park HL, Kim JW, Park CK. Choroidal microvasculature dropout is associated with progressive retinal nerve fiber layer thinning in glaucoma with disc hemorrhage. Ophthalmology. 2018;125(7):1003–13.
64. Rao HL, Sreenivasaiah S, Dixit S, et al. Choroidal microvascular dropout in primary open-angle glaucoma eyes with disc hemorrhage. J Glaucoma. 2019;28(3):181–7.
65. Suh MH, Zangwill LM, Manalastas PIC, et al. Deep-layer microvasculature dropout by optical coherence tomography angiography and microstructure of parapapillary atrophy. Invest Ophthalmol Vis Sci. 2018;59(5):1995–2004.
66. Suh MH, Zangwill LM, Manalastas PI, et al. Deep retinal layer microvasculature dropout detected by the optical coherence tomography angiography in glaucoma. Ophthalmology. 2016;123(12):2509–18.
67. Chihara E, Dimitrova G, Chihara T. Increase in the OCT angiographic peripapillary vessel density by ROCK inhibitor ripasudil instillation: a comparison with brimonidine. Graefes Arch Clin Exp Ophthalmol. 2018;256(7):1257–64.
68. Jiang X, Johnson E, Cepurna W, et al. The effect of age on the response of retinal capillary filling to changes in intraocular pressure measured by optical coherence tomography angiography. Microvasc Res. 2018;115:12–9.
69. Nelson AJ, Chang R, LeTran V, et al. African American Eye Disease Study Group. Invest Ophthalmol Vis Sci. 2019;60(10):3368–73. https://doi.org/10.1167/iovs.19-27035. PMID: 31917454
70. Zhao D, Cho J, Kim MH, et al. Diabetes, fasting glucose, and the risk of glaucoma: a meta-analysis. Ophthalmology. 2015;122(1):72–8.
71. Zhou M, Wang W, Huang W, Zhang X. Diabetes mellitus as a risk factor for open-angle glaucoma: a systematic review and meta-analysis. PLoS One. 2014;9(8):e102972.
72. Marcus MW, de Vries MM, Junoy Montolio FG, Jansonius NM. Myopia as a risk factor for open-angle glaucoma: a systematic review and meta-analysis. Ophthalmology. 2011;118(10):1989–94. e2
73. Lim HB, Kim YW, Kim JM, et al. The importance of signal strength in quantitative assessment of retinal vessel density using optical coherence tomography angiography. Sci Rep. 2018;8(1):12897.
74. Do JL, Sylvester B, Shahidzadeh A, et al. Utility of optical coherence tomography angiography in detecting glaucomatous damage in a uveitic patient with disc congestion: a case report. Am J Ophthalmol Case Rep. 2017;8:78–83.

Examination of the Optic Nerve in Glaucoma

5

Brandon J. Wong, Benjamin Y. Xu, and Mingguang He

Clinical Examination of the Optic Nerve

Examination of the optic nerve remains essential for the diagnosis and management of glaucoma. Despite advances in structural imaging of the optic nerve, the clinical exam is invaluable in identifying glaucomatous optic neuropathy and monitoring patients for signs of progressive disease. The normal optic nerve has a mean vertical disc diameter of 1.88 mm and horizontal disc diameter of 1.77 mm [1]. The mean disc area may vary according to race, with African-Americans reported to have a large disc size compared to other races. Using a variety of methods, estimates of the mean disc area in African-Americans range from 2.14 mm^2 to 3.75 mm^2, 1.7 mm^2 to 2.63 mm^2 in Caucasians, 2.46 mm^2 to 2.67 mm^2 in Hispanics, and 2.47 mm^2 to 3.22 mm^2 in Asians [2]. The size of the optic nerve is best examined after pupillary dilation since examination without dilation leads to significantly poorer interobserver agreement compared to dilated pupils [3]. The optic nerve may be examined in the clinic using a variety of methods, although slit-lamp biomicroscopy is the most commonly employed technique. An accurate estimation of the optic nerve size depends upon the type of high power convex lens used for examination. Correction factors have been proposed for common lenses (+60 D, +78 D, SuperField NC, or +90 D), although a single correction factor for each lens may not be appropriate depending upon the refractive error of the patient [4].

Recording the appearance of the optic nerve with color fundus imaging is critical to document the appearance of the nerve and allows for serial photograph comparisons to evaluate for progression. Fundus imaging is especially beneficial in documenting the presence of an optic disc hemorrhage or a wedge-shaped retinal nerve fiber layer (RNFL) defect. Stereoscopic fundus images are preferable to monoscopic images because monoscopic images have been shown to lead to more interobserver variation and may lead to underestimation of the vertical cup-to-disc ratio (CDR) [5].

The appearance of the optic disc in glaucoma can be quite variable. Classically, four phenotypic appearances of the glaucomatous optic nerve were described: (1) focal localized tissue loss, (2) generalized enlargement of the optic disc cup without localized defect, (3) myopic glaucomatous disc with peripapillary atrophy and tilted discs, and (4) senile sclerotic discs with shallow, saucerized cup and the "moth-eaten appearance" of peripapillary atrophy [6, 7]. The differing

B. J. Wong (✉) · B. Y. Xu
USC Roski Eye Institute, Keck Medicine of University of Southern California, Los Angeles, CA, USA
e-mail: brandon.wong@med.usc.edu

M. He
Department of Ophthalmology, University of Melbourne, Centre for Eye Research Australia, East Melbourne, VIC, Australia

© Springer Nature Switzerland AG 2020
R. Varma et al. (eds.), *Advances in Ocular Imaging in Glaucoma*, Essentials in Ophthalmology, https://doi.org/10.1007/978-3-030-43847-0_5

appearance of the optic disc may be multifactorial and may in part be due to individual variation of the lamina cribrosa and its response to elevated intraocular pressure (IOP) [8].

Clinical Findings of the Optic Nerve in Glaucoma

Optic Nerve Excavation

Excavation of the optic nerve, clinically known as cupping, is the most commonly recognized morphologic change of the glaucomatous optic nerve (Fig. 5.1). The pathophysiology of optic nerve cupping and subsequent optic neuropathy has been researched in experimental monkey studies and has two proposed components: prelaminar thinning and laminar deformation [9]. Prelaminar thinning consists of thinning of the prelaminar tissues due to compression or loss of retinal ganglion cells (RGC) without significant connective tissue involvement. Laminar deformation occurs

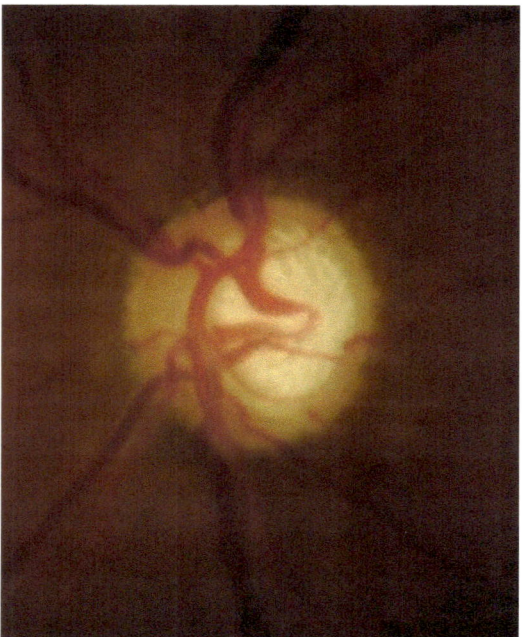

Fig. 5.1 Fundus photograph of the optic nerve demonstrating excavation of the optic nerve with exposure of the laminar pores

as a result of changes of the lamina cribrosa or peripapillary scleral tissues and is thought to be a permanent, IOP-induced change. The laminar component of cupping is predominant in glaucomatous optic neuropathy and is characterized by a posterior displacement of the optic nerve head (ONH) surface [10]. Thus, the defining phenomenon underlying glaucomatous optic neuropathy is deformation and/or remodeling of the neural and connective tissues of the ONH, regardless of the mechanism of injury or the level of IOP [10].

Despite its significant association with glaucoma, optic nerve cupping can also be observed in a number of other optic neuropathies, including methanol toxicity, dominant optic atrophy, optic neuritis, arteritic ischemic optic neuropathy, or intracranial tumors leading to compressive optic neuropathy [11–14].

Optic Nerve Notching

An optic nerve notch is a focal loss of the neural rim width associated with a change in the rim curvature (Fig. 5.2). A notch is indicative of a structural change to the disc as a result of localized glaucomatous damage causing loss of the tissue of the neuroretinal rim.

The Blue Mountains Eye Study found the prevalence of a neural rim notch increased with age, from 2.48% in participants aged <60 years to 4.1% for ages 60–69 years, 7.98% for ages 70–79 years, and 15.3% for ages 80 years or older. A notch was strongly associated with glaucoma diagnosis (OR 21.2, CI 8.8–50.8). The sensitivity and specificity for glaucoma with visual field loss of finding a notch in either eye was 90.3% and 96.8%, respectively. The positive predictive value of a notch was 45.4% and negative predictive value 99.7%.

Peripapillary Atrophy

Peripapillary atrophy (PPA) around the optic nerve is another morphologic finding in the glaucomatous optic nerve. Peripapillary atrophy is more frequently observed in patients with

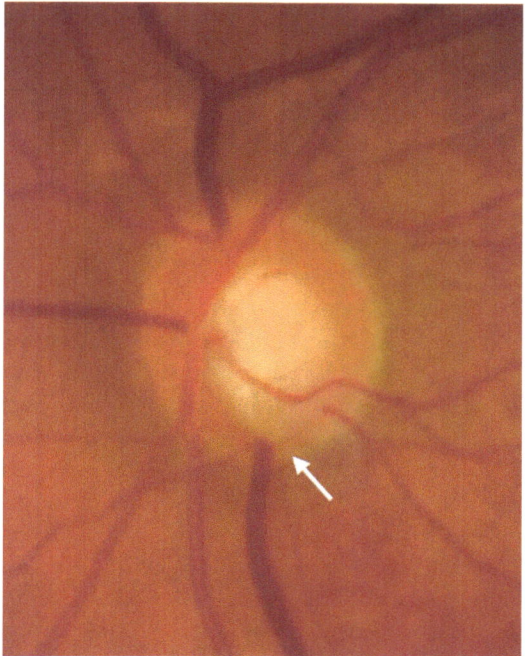

Fig. 5.2 Fundus photograph demonstrating focal notching (white arrow) of the optic nerve at the inferior margin of the neuroretinal rim

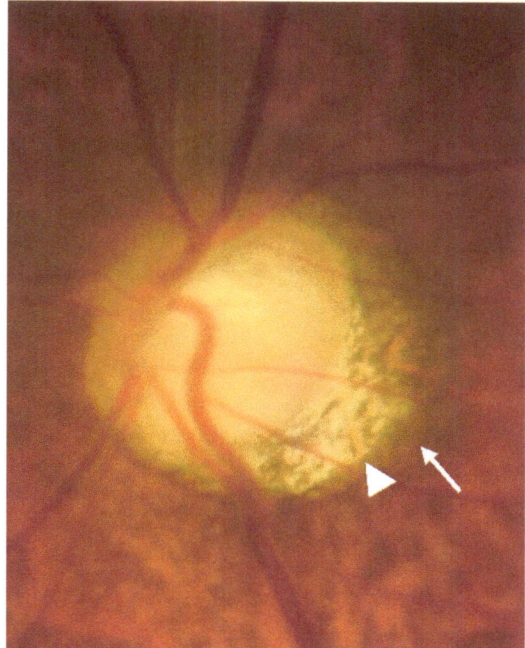

Fig. 5.3 Fundus photograph demonstrating peripapillary atrophy areas of "alpha" zone atrophy (white arrow) and "beta" zone atrophy (white arrowhead)

glaucoma compared to normal patients and is more commonly observed in myopic and older eyes [15]. When compared to PPA in normal eyes, PPA is significantly more extensive in glaucomatous eyes, with more prominent PPA associated with more advanced and chronic disease [16].

Peripapillary atrophy has previously been classified in two different zones: (1) the "alpha" zone located peripherally with irregular hyper- and hypopigmentation and (2) the central "beta" zone with marked atrophy of the choroid and retina revealing the underlying choroidal vessels and sclera [17–19]. Histologically, the "alpha" zone corresponds to pigmentary changes of the retinal pigment epithelium (RPE) while the "beta" zone corresponds to a complete loss of RPE and decreased photoreceptor layer (Fig. 5.3). Accordingly, the "alpha" zone correlates to a relative scotoma on visual field while the "beta" zone relates to an absolute scotoma [17]. The area of peripapillary atrophy, particularly the "beta" zone, has shown significant cor-

relations with neuroretinal rim area, cup-to-disc ratio, nerve fiber layer loss, and mean visual field loss [18]. More recently, a "gamma" zone of peripapillary atrophy, corresponding to the region between the temporal disc margin and the beginning of Bruch's membrane, has been identified histologically and on enhanced depth imaging spectral-domain optical coherence tomography (SD-OCT) [20, 21]. Although the "gamma" zone is associated with longer axial length, longer vertical disc diameter, and old age, it has not been associated with glaucoma [21].

Increasing PPA has been associated with progressive optic nerve damage and progressive glaucomatous visual field loss. In one study, 37% of the eyes showed peripapillary atrophy progression during an 8-year follow-up period. The incidence of PPA progression was significantly higher in eyes with glaucomatous optic disc progression (64%) or glaucomatous visual field progression (75%) compared to eyes without optic disc progression (14%) or glaucomatous visual field progression (25%) [15].

Although PPA can be helpful in determining glaucomatous progression, in comparison to other parameters of the optic disc such as vertical cup-to-disc, total neuroretinal rim area, and rim/disc area ratio, PPA is less useful for differentiating normal from pre-perimetric glaucoma patients. In terms of detecting glaucomatous optic neuropathy, peripapillary atrophy should be considered second order parameter [22]. However, PPA may be helpful in distinguishing glaucomatous from non-glaucomatous optic neuropathy. Studies have shown that PPA does not typically enlarge after non-glaucomatous optic neuropathies such as nonarteritic anterior ischemic optic neuropathy or arteritic anterior ischemic optic neuropathy [23, 24].

Disc Hemorrhage

Optic disc hemorrhages (DH) are characterized by flame-shaped or splinter-shaped hemorrhages located in the retinal nerve fiber layer at the level of the neuroretinal rim or immediately adjacent to the optic disc margin (Fig. 5.4). Disc hemorrhage is not a specific entity to glaucoma and

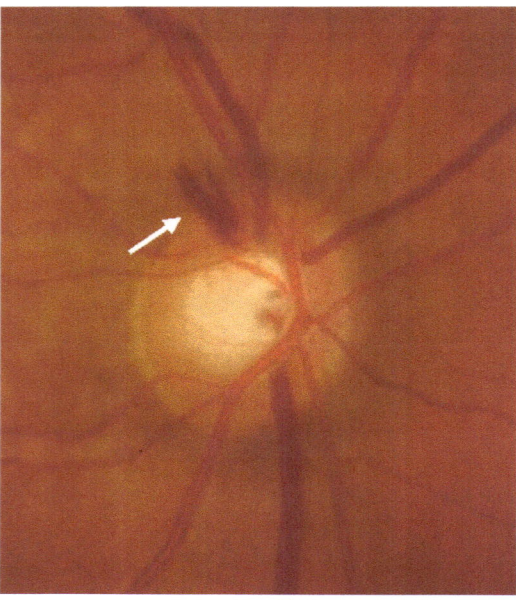

Fig. 5.4 Fundus photograph demonstrating superior disc hemorrhage of the optic nerve (white arrow)

can occur in a number of other ocular conditions, including retinal vascular disease such as diabetic retinopathy or vascular occlusion, posterior vitreous detachment, ischemic optic neuropathy, or optic disc drusen. Jannik P. Bjerrum is credited with first reporting the association with DH and glaucoma in 1889 [25].

Although the exact mechanism of DH has not been definitively established, both mechanical and vascular factors appear to be involved in the pathogenesis. The mechanical theory proposes DH are caused by degenerative changes of the connective tissue causing microvascular damage, specifically small blood vessel rupture at the level of the lamina cribrosa at the optic disc margin or RNFL defect [1, 26]. With the advent of enhanced depth imaging spectral-domain optical coherence tomography (SD-OCT), structural alterations of the lamina have been strongly associated with disc hemorrhage. Several studies have reported higher percentage of lamina cribrosa-structural alteration or disinsertion in POAG eyes with disc hemorrhage than those without [27, 28]. These laminar changes have been correlated spatially with the location of DH, suggesting microvascular damage may result from a structural lamina change near its insertion [29]. The vascular theory arises from the association of disc hemorrhage with systemic vascular disorders or dysfunctional vascular autoregulation around the optic nerve head [30]. Vascular risk factors for disc hemorrhage have previously been identified; one randomized, double-masked, multicenter clinical trial examining low-tension glaucoma patients found that migraine, baseline narrower neuroretinal rim width, low-systolic blood pressure, mean arterial ocular perfusion pressure, and use of systemic beta blockers were significant risk factors for disc hemorrhage [31].

Disc hemorrhages are more commonly seen in patients with glaucoma than in those with OHTN and are more frequent in so-called normal-tension glaucoma compared to high-tension glaucoma [32]. In cross-sectional studies, the prevalence of DH varies, ranging from 0% to 0.4% in normal eyes, 0.4–10% in OHTN eyes, 4.2–17.6% in eyes with high-tension glaucoma, and 20.5–33.3% in eyes with normal-tension glaucoma [33–36]. In the 13-year follow-up of patients in the Ocular Hypertension Treatment Study (OHTS), DH was found to be an independent predictive factor for development of POAG in patients with OHTN. The cumulative incidence of POAG in eyes with DH was 25.6% compared to 12.9% in eyes without DH, and the presence of DH during follow-up increased the risk of developing POAG 2.6-fold [33]. The OHTS trial also showed the cumulative incidence of optic disc hemorrhage was 0.5% per year prior to the development of glaucoma and 2.5% per year after development of glaucoma [37]. Interestingly, the majority of eyes (78%) with DH did not progress to glaucoma over a median follow-up of 49 months after DH.

Multiple studies of eyes with DH have shown significantly faster rate of visual field (VF) progression [38–40]. Both the Collaborative Normal-Tension Glaucoma Study and the Early Manifest Glaucoma Trial (EMGT) demonstrated that glaucomatous eyes with DH had significantly more visual field progression than eyes without DH [41, 42]. One study showed the overall rate of visual field index (VFI) change in eyes with hemorrhages was significantly faster than in eyes without hemorrhages (−0.88%/year vs. −0.38%/year) [40]. In addition to deterioration of the overall VF, DH can lead to spatially consistent and localized VF loss. Interestingly, this localized VF loss can be observed in regions prior to the development of a DH and can continue to progress in the same regions at a faster rate after DH occurrence [39]. This finding suggests that rapid, localized disease progression may predispose to formation of DH and progressive VF loss continues secondary to ongoing damage at or near this location.

The role of IOP-lowering therapy in the setting of DH without additional evidence of glaucomatous progression remains controversial. The Early Manifest Glaucoma Trial reported that after a median follow-up of 8 years, patients with newly diagnosed glaucoma started on IOP-lowering therapy did not have a significant difference in the presence or frequency of DH compared to patients who were observed with no therapy [42]. Using event-based analysis for visual field progression, the authors found DH were associated with time to progression, but there was no interaction between treatment group and DH. In contrast, a study using trend-based analysis reported the difference in rates of visual field loss pre- and post-disc hemorrhage was significantly related to the reduction of IOP in the post-hemorrhage period compared with the pre-hemorrhage period. Each 1 mmHg of IOP reduction was associated with a difference of 0.31%/year in the rate of VFI change [40].

DH have also been associated with structural progression in glaucoma. Localized thinning of the RNFL has been reported after DH detection in patients with glaucoma [43–45]. One study found that after mean 38 months of follow-up, 72.7% of eyes in the DH group showed OCT-determined progression on a clock-hour basis compared with 27.3% of the fellow eyes in the non-DH group [43]. Focal rim notching may precede the occurrence of a disc hemorrhage at or adjacent to the notch [46].

A clinical examination of the disc at every visit should include a documentation of disc hemorrhage, especially since DH may not be visualized by other optic nerve imaging modalities. The presence of DH should be documented with fundus photographs to monitor for resolution, although the vast majority of DH may take 4 weeks or more to resolve [34]. The presence of a DH on examination should spur the clinician to be more vigilant for signs of glaucomatous progression, with careful consideration of more frequent monitoring and possible institution or escalation of medical therapy.

Cup-to-Disc Enlargement and Disc Asymmetry

Enlargement of the vertical cup-to-disc ratio (VCDR) is a well-documented indicator of the glaucomatous optic nerve (Fig. 5.5). One study reported that the prevalence of disc-defined glaucoma in one or both eyes was 1.6% among patients with VCDR <0.60 compared to a prevalence of 31.4% in patients with VCDR ≥0.6 [47]. Besides examining the optic nerve for changes in

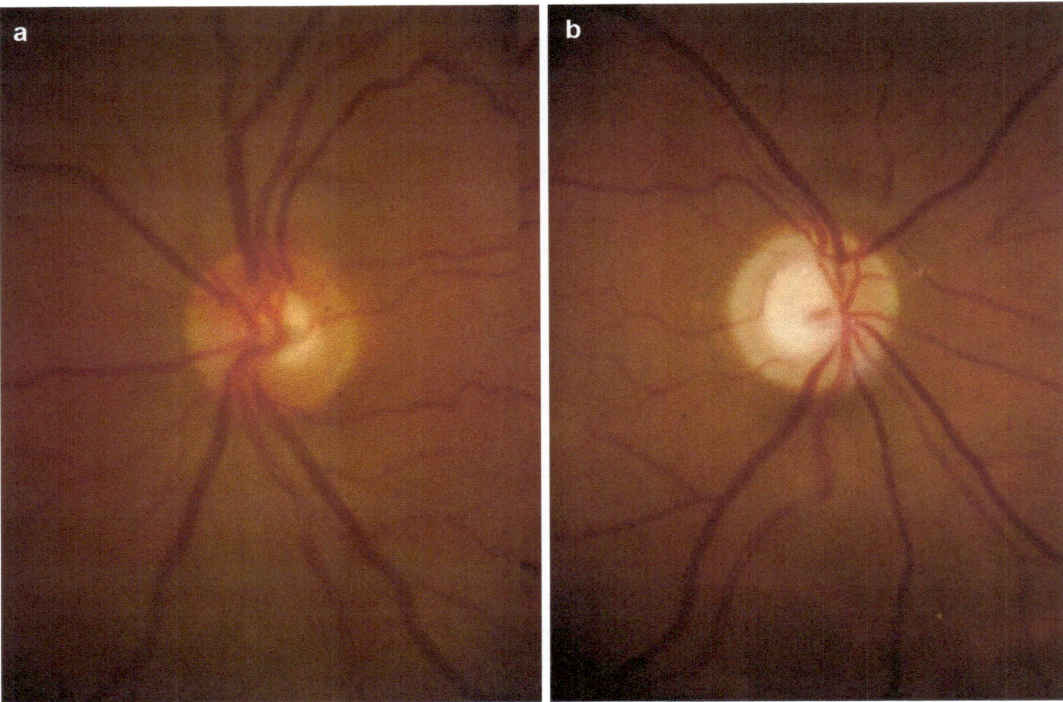

Fig. 5.5 Fundus photographs of the right (**a**) and left (**b**) eyes of a patient demonstrating asymmetry of the cup-to-disc ratio

the VCDR, it is important to compare the VCDR in the fellow eye for signs of asymmetry as a significant amount of VCDR is suggestive of glaucoma (Fig. 5.5) [48]. Some amount of VCDR asymmetry can be found in normal patients, especially older patients. In a study looking at US adults from the National Health and Nutrition Examination Survey (NHANES), VCDR asymmetry ≥ 0.20 occurred in approximately 2% of adults without glaucoma [49]. The same study reported the odds of VCDR asymmetry ≥ 0.20 were 1.44 times higher per 10-year increase in age. Each 0.10 increase in VCDR asymmetry was associated with a 2.57 times higher adjusted odds of disc plus field defined glaucoma. The positive predictive value (PPV) for disc plus field defined that glaucoma for VCDR asymmetry ≥ 0.20 was 7.0%, and when VCDR asymmetry cutoff was increased to ≥ 0.30, the PPV increases to 37.7%. Based on this study, VCDR asymmetry may be physiologic in many patients, and given the low PPV even at high degrees of asymmetry, it may

be a poor measure for diagnosing glaucoma in isolation. Nonetheless, a VCDR >0.3 may be sufficient to initiate a further diagnostic workup and to identify individuals who may be at high risk for glaucoma. The size of the optic nerve should always be considered when evaluating the VCDR since larger optic nerves have a larger VCDR.

Retinal Blood Vessel Changes

Characteristics changes to the central or paracentral retinal blood vessels around the nerve can also be observed in the glaucomatous optic nerve [50–52]. Displacement of the central retinal vessels has been termed "nasalization of the blood vessels"; however, the change to the blood vessels may better be described as a centrifugal displacement of the vessels away from the center of the optic disc occurring over time (Fig. 5.6) [52]. Retinal blood vessel (RBV) shifts have been associated with functionally progressive glau-

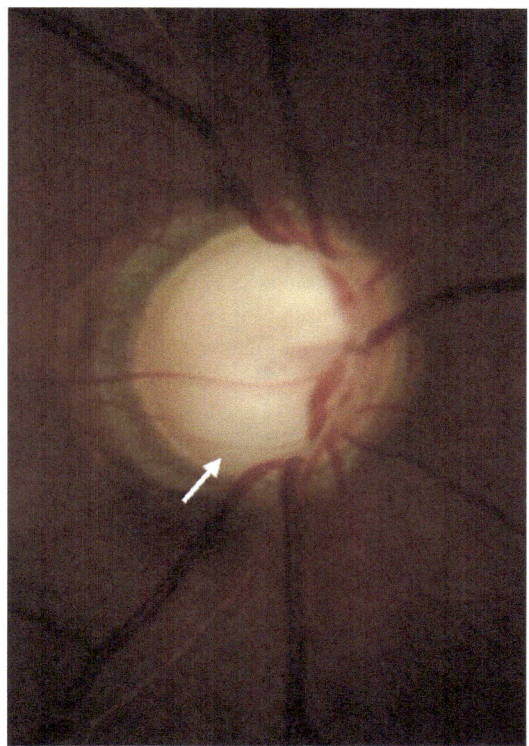

Fig. 5.6 Fundus photograph demonstrating nasalization of the central retinal vessels and inferior baring of a circumlinear vessel (white arrow)

coma. One study examined serial photographs of the nerve using an automated alternation flicker technique to identify discrete positional shifts in the RBV. They found that RBV shifts were noted in 33 of 125 (26.4%) longitudinally followed glaucomatous eyes, and RBV shifts were present in 12.1% of minimal progressors versus 31.5% of moderate and fast progressors. The rate of VF progression was statistically associated with RBV shift [53]. Other changes such as "bayoneting" of vessels or "baring" of the circumlinear vessels has also been described in glaucomatous eyes. "Bayoneting" of vessels refers to the sharp bend or kink of blood vessels as they cross the edge of the optic cup, most easily seen with larger blood vessels. Circumlinear vessels are blood vessels (arteries or veins) that follow the physiologic disc margin either above or below the central vessel trunk. "Baring" of these vessels refers to their displacement posteriorly to the

bottom or the side wall of the optic cup and is thought to occur as a result of enlargement of the cup [54]. While "baring" of circumlinear vessels may be frequently present in glaucomatous eyes, it can be seen in other causes of optic atrophy and should not be considered as a specific sign or predictor of glaucomatous damage [51, 54].

Future Directions: Optic Disc Evaluation and Deep Learning

One emerging area in ophthalmic diagnostic imaging is the use of artificial intelligence (AI) models that utilize automated computer programs equipped with deep learning algorithms. Deep learning (DL) is a category of artificial intelligence referring to the use of automated systems to independently improve upon tasks, such as decision-making or feature recognition, without specific expert knowledge guiding its actions [55]. These algorithms can use a wide variety of input data, categorize the data, and create an output leading to a classification decision (i.e., disease or no disease, progression or no progression). In practice, the algorithms can be "supervised" or "unsupervised." "Supervised" algorithms are automated programs that depend upon a clinical reference standard or "ground truth" data set defined by a human. For example, an algorithm may use computer vision interpretation of labelled images to learn features from a reference data set and then apply its knowledge to a separate test data set for validation. In contrast, "unsupervised" DL may take raw input data, without any human expert standard, and categorize the information into classifications that may or may not coincide with human standards.

DL algorithms have already been used to identify diabetic retinopathy and macular edema with excellent sensitivity and specificity [56, 57]. DL systems with varying algorithms have been used to detect glaucomatous optic neuropathy based on color fundus photographs [58–60]. The algorithms may be based on segmentation methods or non-segmentation methods. Initial studies using automated systems utilized feature extraction (a segmentation method) in which the system would analyze fundus images and extract topographic features of the optic disc, such as CDR, neural rim width, presence of PPA, and RNFL defects. Using feature extraction, one study examined 2252 fundus photos and found an area under receiver (AUC) operating characteristic curve of 0.792 with a sensitivity of 71.6% and specificity of 71.7% for detecting glaucoma [59]. Using segmentation methods such as feature extraction may introduce segmentation and misalignment error into the system that could potentially lead to misclassification. Combining feature extraction with deep convolutional networks derived from large-scale data sets may improve glaucoma detection. One study by Li et al. using this combination of holistic and local feature method found an AUC of 0.838, similar to that of manual detection of glaucoma [60]. In another study by Li et al., instead of using feature extraction technology, the DL algorithm used a non-segmentation method looking at global labeled images from 48,116 fundus photos to learn predictive features [58]. In this study, the DL algorithm identified referable glaucomatous optic neuropathy with a sensitivity of 95.6% and specificity of 92.0%. Physiologic cupping and pathologic/high myopia were the most common cause of false positives. The most common causes of false-negative results were coexisting eye conditions, specifically pathologic/high myopia, diabetic retinopathy, and age-related macular degeneration.

Two recent studies by Thompson and Medeiros out of Duke University have trained DL algorithms to evaluate fundus photographs to provide objective and quantitative data regarding glaucomatous neural loss. One inherent limitation of a machine's learning ability is the training process by which it learns how to correctly classify or make predictions. Instead of using a subjectively graded fundus photos by humans as reference standard to teach the machine, these studies use objective data, such as that obtained from SD-OCT, to train a DL network. The first study used a DL algorithm to predict SD-OCT RNFL thickness from assessment of optic disc photographs [61]. The authors examined 32,820 pairs of optic disc photographs and SD-OCT

RNFL scans from 1198 patients. The DL algorithm prediction of average RNFL thickness from all 6292 optic disc photographs in the test set was 83.3 ± 14.5 mm, whereas the mean average RNFL thickness from all corresponding SD-OCT scans was 82.5 ± 16.8 mm ($P = 0.164$). There was a strong correlation between predicted and observed RNFL thickness with mean absolute error of the predictions of 7.39 mm. The AUC curves for discriminating glaucomatous from healthy eyes with the DL predictions and actual SD-OCT average RNFL thickness measurements were 0.944 (95% confidence interval [CI], 0.912–0.966) and 0.940 (95% CI, 0.902–0.966), respectively. The second study used a similar DL algorithm to predict the relativity to the Bruch's membrane opening minimum rim width (BMO-MRW) and compare the results to actual SD-OCT measurements [62]. Overall, 9282 pairs of optic disc photographs and SD-OCT optic nerve head scans were used. The algorithm predictions of global BMO-MRW from all optic disc photographs in the test set were highly correlated with the observed values from SD-OCT, with mean absolute error of the predictions of 27.8 mm. The AUC for discriminating glaucomatous eyes from healthy eyes with the DL predictions and actual SD-OCT global BMO-MRW measurements were 0.945 (95% confidence interval [CI]: 0.874–0.980) and 0.933 (95% CI: 0.856–0.975). Using the BMO-MRW to distinguish glaucoma eyes from normal eyes may be helpful in cases of high myopia, in which subjective graders tend to underdiagnose glaucoma. There are several advantages of using this type of DL algorithm. One advantage is that it does not depend upon subjective human grading of fundus photographs to determine glaucomatous damage. Optic disc grading by expert humans has varying degrees of reliability and is inherently subjective [5, 63]. Using a machine, such as SD-OCT, which has been shown to provide objective and reproducible data of the optic nerve in glaucoma, eliminates this issue of subjectivity and avoids the time-consuming nature of grading fundus photos. Another advantage of the DL algorithm is its ability to detect longitudinal changes over time. Prior studies using DL algorithms have used a binary output (yes-no) to classify fundus photographs as glaucomatous or normal. By incorporating continuous data such as RNFL thickness or BMO-MRW in the algorithm, future DL programs could potentially be used to monitor glaucoma or identify progression.

While the use of DL in glaucoma is still in its nascent stages, the promise of more efficient and more objective methods to identify glaucomatous disease or predict damage is fascinating. Using automated methods to detect glaucoma would have tremendous value to screening programs in remote locations or in populations with a shortage of trained professionals. Future studies using large-scale data sets will help to clarify which type of deep learning algorithms are most accurate and reliable.

Compliance with Ethical Requirements Brandon J. Wong, Benjamin Y. Xu, and Mingguang He declare that they have no conflict of interest. No human or animal studies were carried out by the authors of this chapter.

References

1. Quigley HA, Brown AE, Morrison JD, Drance SM. The size and shape of the optic disc in normal human eyes. Arch Ophthalmol (Chicago, Ill 1960). 1990;108(1):51–7.
2. Hoffmann EM, Zangwill LM, Crowston JG, Weinreb RN. Optic disk size and glaucoma. Surv Ophthalmol. 2007;52(1):32–49. https://doi.org/10.1016/j.survophthal.2006.10.002.
3. Kirwan JF, Gouws P, Linnell AE, Crowston J, Bunce C. Pharmacological mydriasis and optic disc examination. Br J Ophthalmol. 2000;84(8):894–8.
4. Ansari-Shahrezaei S, Maar N, Biowski R, Stur M. Biomicroscopic measurement of the optic disc with a high-power positive lens. Invest Ophthalmol Vis Sci. 2001;42(1):153–7.
5. Varma R, Steinmann WC, Scott IU. Expert agreement in evaluating the optic disc for glaucoma. Ophthalmology. 1992;99(2):215–21.
6. Geijssen HC, Greve EL. The spectrum of primary open angle glaucoma. I: Senile sclerotic glaucoma versus high tension glaucoma. Ophthalmic Surg. 1987;18(3):207–13.
7. Geijssen H, Greve E. Focal ischaemic normal pressure glaucoma versus high pressure glaucoma. Doc Ophthalmol. 1990;75(3–4):291–301.
8. Sawada Y, Hangai M, Murata K, Ishikawa M, Yoshitomi T. Lamina cribrosa depth variation measured by spectral-domain optical coherence tomography within and between four glaucomatous optic disc phenotypes.

Investig Ophthalmol Vis Sci. 2015;56(10):5777–84. https://doi.org/10.1167/iovs.14-15942.
9. Yang H, Reynaud J, Lockwood H, et al. The connective tissue phenotype of glaucomatous cupping in the monkey eye – Clinical and research implications. Prog Retin Eye Res. 2017;59:1–52. https://doi.org/10.1016/j.preteyeres.2017.03.001.
10. Burgoyne C. The morphological difference between glaucoma and other optic neuropathies. J Neuroophthalmol. 2015;35 Suppl 1:S8–S21. https://doi.org/10.1097/WNO.0000000000000289.
11. Danesh-Meyer HV, Savino PJ, Sergott RC. The prevalence of cupping in end-stage arteritic and nonarteritic anterior ischemic optic neuropathy. Ophthalmology. 2001;108(3):593–8.
12. Bianchi-Marzoli S, Rizzo JF, Brancato R, Lessell S. Quantitative analysis of optic disc cupping in compressive optic neuropathy. Ophthalmology. 1995;102(3):436–40.
13. Rebolleda G, Noval S, Contreras I, Arnalich-Montiel F, García-Perez JL, Muñoz-Negrete FJ. Optic disc cupping after optic neuritis evaluated with optic coherence tomography. Eye (Lond). 2009;23(4):890–4. https://doi.org/10.1038/eye.2008.117.
14. Fournier AV, Damji KF, Epstein DL, Pollock SC. Disc excavation in dominant optic atrophy: differentiation from normal tension glaucoma. Ophthalmology. 2001;108(9):1595–602.
15. Uchida H, Ugurlu S, Caprioli J. Increasing peripapillary atrophy is associated with progressive glaucoma. Ophthalmology. 1998;105(8):1541–5. https://doi.org/10.1016/S0161-6420(98)98044-7.
16. Wilensky JT, Kolker AE. Peripapillary changes in glaucoma. Am J Ophthalmol. 1976;81(3):341–5.
17. Jonas JB. Clinical implications of peripapillary atrophy in glaucoma. Curr Opin Ophthalmol. 2005;16(2):84–8. https://doi.org/10.1097/01.icu.0000156135.20570.30.
18. Jonas JB, Fernández MC, Naumann GO. Glaucomatous parapapillary atrophy. Occurrence and correlations. Arch Ophthalmol (Chicago, Ill 1960). 1992;110(2):214–22.
19. Jonas JB, Naumann GO. Parapapillary chorioretinal atrophy in normal and glaucoma eyes. II. Correlations. Invest Ophthalmol Vis Sci. 1989;30(5):919–26.
20. Jonas JB, Jonas SB, Jonas RA, et al. Parapapillary atrophy: histological gamma zone and delta zone. PLoS One. 2017;7:e47237. https://doi.org/10.1371/journal.pone.0047237.
21. Dai Y, Jonas JB, Huang H, Wang M, Sun X. Microstructure of parapapillary atrophy: beta zone and gamma zone. Invest Ophthalmol Vis Sci. 2013;54(3):2013–8. https://doi.org/10.1167/iovs.12-11255.
22. Jonas JB, Bergua A, Schmitz-Valckenberg P, Papastathopoulos KI, Budde WM. Ranking of optic disc variables for detection of glaucomatous optic nerve damage. Invest Ophthalmol Vis Sci. 2000;41(7):1764–73.
23. Rath EZ, Rehany U, Linn S, Rumelt S. Correlation between optic disc atrophy and aetiology: anterior

ischaemic optic neuropathy vs optic neuritis. Eye (Lond). 2003;17(9):1019–24. https://doi.org/10.1038/sj.eye.6700691.

24. Hayreh SS, Jonas JB. Optic disc morphology after arteritic anterior ischemic optic neuropathy. Ophthalmology. 2001;108(9):1586–94.

25. Bjerrum J. Om en Tilfojelse til den Saedvanlige Synsfelfundersogelse samt om Synfelet ved Glaukom. Nord Ophthalmol Tskr (Copenh). 1889;2:141–85.

26. Nitta K, Sugiyama K, Higashide T, Ohkubo S, Tanahashi T, Kitazawa Y. Does the enlargement of retinal nerve fiber layer defects relate to disc hemorrhage or progressive visual field loss in normal-tension glaucoma? J Glaucoma. 2011;20(3):189–95. https://doi.org/10.1097/IJG.0b013e3181e0799c.

27. Sharpe GP, Danthurebandara VM, Vianna JR, et al. Optic disc hemorrhages and laminar disinsertions in glaucoma. Ophthalmology. 2016;123(9):1949–56. https://doi.org/10.1016/j.ophtha.2016.06.001.

28. Kim YK, Park KH. Lamina cribrosa defects in eyes with glaucomatous disc haemorrhage. Acta Ophthalmol. 2016;94(6):e468–73. https://doi.org/10.1111/aos.12903.

29. Lee EJ, Kim T-W, Kim M, Girard MJA, Mari JM, Weinreb RN. Recent structural alteration of the peripheral lamina cribrosa near the location of disc hemorrhage in glaucoma. Invest Ophthalmol Vis Sci. 2014;55(4):2805–15. https://doi.org/10.1167/iovs.13-12742.

30. Kim YW, Jeoung JW, Kim YK, Park KH. Clinical implications of in vivo lamina cribrosa imaging in glaucoma. J Glaucoma. 2017;26(9):753–61. https://doi.org/10.1097/IJG.0000000000000728.

31. Furlanetto RL, De Moraes CG, Teng CC, et al. Risk factors for optic disc hemorrhage in the low-pressure glaucoma treatment study. Am J Ophthalmol. 2014;157(5):945–952.e1. https://doi.org/10.1016/j.ajo.2014.02.009.

32. Gloster J. Incidence of optic disc haemorrhages in chronic simple glaucoma and ocular hypertension. Br J Ophthalmol. 1981;65(7):452–6.

33. Budenz DL, Huecker JB, Gedde SJ, Gordon M, Kass M, Ocular Hypertension Treatment Study Group. Thirteen-year follow-up of optic disc hemorrhages in the ocular hypertension treatment study. Am J Ophthalmol. 2017;174:126–33. https://doi.org/10.1016/j.ajo.2016.10.023.

34. Kitazawa Y, Shirato S, Yamamoto T. Optic disc hemorrhage in low-tension glaucoma. Ophthalmology. 1986;93(6):853–7.

35. Suh MH, Park KH. Period prevalence and incidence of optic disc haemorrhage in normal tension glaucoma and primary open-angle glaucoma. Clin Exp Ophthalmol. 2011;39(6):513–9. https://doi.org/10.1111/j.1442-9071.2010.02482.x.

36. Healey P. Optic disc haemorrhage: the more we look the more we find. Clin Exp Ophthalmol. 2011;39(6):485–6. https://doi.org/10.1111/j.1442-9071.2011.02648.x.

37. Budenz DL, Anderson DR, Feuer WJ, et al. Detection and prognostic significance of optic disc hemorrhages during the ocular hypertension treatment study. Ophthalmology. 2006;113(12):6. https://doi.org/10.1016/j.ophtha.2006.06.022.

38. Kim JM, Kyung H, Azarbod P, Lee JM, Caprioli J. Disc haemorrhage is associated with the fast component, but not the slow component, of visual field decay rate in glaucoma. Br J Ophthalmol. 2014;98(11):1555–9. https://doi.org/10.1136/bjophthalmol-2013-304584.

39. De Moraes CGV, Prata TS, Liebmann CA, Tello C, Ritch R, Liebmann JM. Spatially consistent, localized visual field loss before and after disc haemorrhage. Investig Opthalmol Vis Sci. 2009;50(10):4727. https://doi.org/10.1167/iovs.09-3446.

40. Medeiros FA, Alencar LM, Sample PA, Zangwill LM, Susanna R, Weinreb RN. The relationship between intraocular pressure reduction and rates of progressive visual field loss in eyes with optic disc hemorrhage. Ophthalmology. 2010;117(11):2061–6. https://doi.org/10.1016/j.ophtha.2010.02.015.

41. Drance S, Anderson DR, Schulzer M, Collaborative Normal-Tension Glaucoma Study Group. Risk factors for progression of visual field abnormalities in normal-tension glaucoma. Am J Ophthalmol. 2001;131(6):699–708.

42. Bengtsson B, Leske MC, Yang Z, Heijl A, EMGT Group. Disc hemorrhages and treatment in the early manifest glaucoma trial. Ophthalmology. 2008;115(11):2044–8. https://doi.org/10.1016/j.ophtha.2008.05.031.

43. Suh MH, Park KH, Kim H, et al. Glaucoma progression after the first-detected optic disc hemorrhage by optical coherence tomography. J Glaucoma. 2012;21(6):358–66. https://doi.org/10.1097/IJG.0b013e3182120700.

44. Choi F, Park KH, Kim DM, Kim TW. Retinal nerve fiber layer thickness evaluation using optical coherence tomography in eyes with optic disc hemorrhage. Ophthalmic Surg Lasers Imaging. 2007;38(2):118–25.

45. Hwang YH, Kim YY, Kim HK, Sohn YH. Changes in retinal nerve fiber layer thickness after optic disc hemorrhage in glaucomatous eyes. J Glaucoma. 2014;23(8):547–52. https://doi.org/10.1097/IJG.0000000000000083.

46. Law SK, Choe R, Caprioli J. Optic disk characteristics before the occurrence of disk hemorrhage in glaucoma patients. Am J Ophthalmol. 2001;132(3):411–3.

47. Boland MV, Gupta P, Ko F, Zhao D, Guallar E, Friedman DS. Evaluation of frequency-doubling technology perimetry as a means of screening for glaucoma and other eye diseases using the national health and nutrition examination survey. JAMA Ophthalmol. 2016;134(1):57–62. https://doi.org/10.1001/jamaophthalmol.2015.4459.

48. Fishman RS. Optic disc asymmetry. A sign of ocular hypertension. Arch Ophthalmol (Chicago, Ill 1960). 1970;84(5):590–4.

49. Qiu M, Boland MV, Ramulu PY. Cup-to-disc ratio asymmetry in U.S. adults: prevalence and association with glaucoma in the 2005–2008 National Health and Nutrition Examination Survey. Ophthalmology. 2017;124(8):1229–36. https://doi.org/10.1016/j.ophtha.2017.03.049.

50. Armaly MF. The optic cup in the normal eye. I. Cup width, depth, vessel displacement, ocular tension and outflow facility. Am J Ophthalmol. 1969;68(3):401–7.

51. Osher RH, Herschler J. The significance of baring of the circumlinear vessel. A prospective study. Arch Ophthalmol (Chicago, Ill 1960). 1981;99(5):817–8.

52. Varma R, Spaeth GL, Hanau C, Steinmann WC, Feldman RM. Positional changes in the vasculature of the optic disk in glaucoma. Am J Ophthalmol. 1987;104(5):457–64.

53. Radcliffe NM, Smith SD, Syed ZA, et al. Retinal blood vessel positional shifts and glaucoma progression. Ophthalmology. 2014;121(4):842–8. https://doi.org/10.1016/j.ophtha.2013.11.002.

54. Sutton GE, Motolko MA, Phelps CD. Baring of a circumlinear vessel in glaucoma. Arch Ophthalmol. 1983;101(5):739–44. https://doi.org/10.1001/archopht.1983.01040010739007.

55. Zheng C, Johnson TV, Garg A, Boland MV. Artificial intelligence in glaucoma. Curr Opin Ophthalmol. 2019;30(2):97–103. https://doi.org/10.1097/ICU.0000000000000552.

56. Gargeya R, Leng T. Automated identification of diabetic retinopathy using deep learning. Ophthalmology. 2017;124(7):962–9. https://doi.org/10.1016/j.ophtha.2017.02.008.

57. Gulshan V, Peng L, Coram M, et al. Development and validation of a deep learning algorithm for detection of diabetic retinopathy in retinal fundus photographs. JAMA. 2016;316(22):2402–10. https://doi.org/10.1001/jama.2016.17216.

58. Li Z, He Y, Keel S, Meng W, Chang RT, He M. Efficacy of a deep learning system for detecting glaucomatous optic neuropathy based on color fundus photographs. Ophthalmology. 2018;125(8):1199–206. https://doi.org/10.1016/j.ophtha.2018.01.023.

59. Chakrabarty L, Joshi GD, Chakravarty A, Raman GV, Krishnadas SR, Sivaswamy J. Automated detection of glaucoma from topographic features of the optic nerve head in color fundus photographs. J Glaucoma. 2016;25(7):590–7. https://doi.org/10.1097/IJG.0000000000000354.

60. Li A, Cheng J, Wong DWK, Liu J. Integrating holistic and local deep features for glaucoma classification. Proc Annu Int Conf IEEE Eng Med Biol Soc EMBS. 2016;2016-Octob:1328–31. https://doi.org/10.1109/EMBC.2016.7590952.

61. Medeiros FA, Jammal AA, Thompson AC. From machine to machine: an OCT-trained deep learning algorithm for objective quantification of glaucomatous damage in fundus photographs. Ophthalmology. 2019;126(4):513–21. https://doi.org/10.1016/j.ophtha.2018.12.033.

62. Thompson AC, Jammal AA, Medeiros FA. A deep learning algorithm to quantify neuroretinal rim loss from optic disc photographs. Am J Ophthalmol. 2019;201(Dl):9–18. https://doi.org/10.1016/j.ajo.2019.01.011.

63. Tielsch JM, Katz J, Quigley HA, Miller NR, Sommer A. Intraobserver and interobserver agreement in measurement of optic disc characteristics. Ophthalmology. 1988;95(3):350–6.

Ultrasound in the Management of Glaucoma

6

Jiun L. Do, Youmin He, Yueqiao Qu, Qifa Zhou, and Zhongping Chen

Summary

Echography remains an important diagnostic tool for glaucoma despite the development of optics-based imaging modalities such as anterior segment optical coherence tomography (AS-OCT). Conventional ultrasound with a 10 MHz B-scan probe allows for reliable visualization of the posterior segment of the eye. With high-frequency 35–100 MHz B-scan probes, ultrasound biomicroscopy (UBM) expands the clinical versatility of ultrasound, providing higher-resolution images of the anterior segment but with reduced depth of tissue penetration from shorter wavelength sound waves [1]. While AS-OCT is able to acquire images of higher spatial resolution than UBM with less dependence on operator experience, ultrasound continues to be relevant in the clinical management of glaucoma as sound waves are unaffected by media opacities that would otherwise preclude optical evaluation techniques and also allows for the visualization of anatomical structures posterior to the iris, including the ciliary body. This chapter will cover the clinical applications of ultrasound in evaluating various types of glaucoma and the complications following glaucoma surgeries. It will also provide information on recent research using ultrasound to assess the biomechanical properties of ocular structures related to glaucoma.

Ultrasound Instrumentation

Ultrasound information may be acquired by a one-dimensional echograph (A-scan) or as a two-dimensional acoustic section (B-scan, UBM). An A-scan can be used to ascertain the axial length of the eye. In cases of ocular lesions, an A-scan can provide quantitative echography including information on reflectivity, internal structure, and sound attenuation, which correlate with the histopathology of certain lesions.

Acquisition of B-scans should include axial, transverse, and longitudinal scans to be a complete examination. One of the initial indications for the use of ultrasound in glaucoma was to assess the optic cup size in eyes with opaque media [2]. Direct visualization of the optic nerve is the gold standard in the evaluation of the glau-

J. L. Do
Shiley Eye Institute, Department of Ophthalmology, University of California San Diego, La Jolla, CA, USA

Y. He · Y. Qu · Z. Chen (✉)
Department of Biomedical Engineering and Beckman Laser Institute, University of California, Irvine, Irvine, CA, USA
e-mail: z2chen@uci.edu

Q. Zhou
Department of Ophthalmology, Keck School of Medicine of University of Southern California, Los Angeles, CA, USA

Department of Biomedical Engineering, University of Southern California, Los Angeles, CA, USA

© Springer Nature Switzerland AG 2020
R. Varma et al. (eds.), *Advances in Ocular Imaging in Glaucoma*, Essentials in Ophthalmology,
https://doi.org/10.1007/978-3-030-43847-0_6

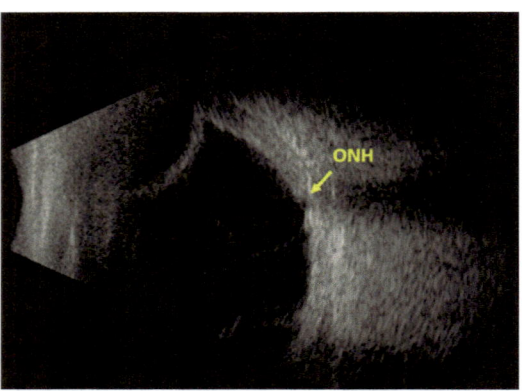

Fig. 6.1 Axial B-scan image of an eye with severe glaucoma showing advanced cupping of the optic nerve head (ONH). Peripheral choroidal effusions are also present secondary to low intraocular pressures following glaucoma surgery

coma and is necessary to detect physiological findings such as disc hemorrhages, parapapillary atrophy, cupping, and bayonetting. However, in cases of media opacities that obscure the ability to visualize the optic disc, ultrasound is reliably able to detect large cups. Shallow or saucershaped cups are less reliably able to be categorized (Fig. 6.1) [2].

With immersion B-scan, evaluation of the anterior segment is also possible but does not provide the resolution of UBM. UBM scans at the corneal limbus provide high-resolution images of the anterior segment and of structures posterior to the iris. Combining these various ultrasound modalities in the clinical setting assist in the evaluation and management of various forms of glaucoma.

Childhood Glaucoma

The diagnosis of childhood glaucoma relies on the findings of elevated intraocular pressure (IOP), reproducible visual field defects, increased eye size, changes in the cornea or corneal diameter, and/or glaucomatous optic nerve findings [3]. Axial length as determined by ultrasound biometry directly correlates with the diagnostic criterion of eye size. Additionally, the positive correlation between the axial length and IOP can

be indicative of the adequacy of glaucoma treatments as long-standing IOP elevations can lead to elongation of the eye beyond normal growth [4]. In myopic eyes, the differentiation between normal growth and glaucomatous changes can be difficult; however, enlargement of the eye secondary to congenital glaucoma is associated with increasing anterior chamber depth and decreasing lens thickness [5].

Pigment Dispersion Glaucoma

Contact between zonular fibers and the posterior iris pigment epithelium releases pigment granules that may lead to the development of pigment dispersion glaucoma. Posterior bowing of the iris ("reverse pupillary block") results in greater contact between the iris and zonular fibers [6]. Imaging of the iris with UBM is able to provide information regarding the concave iris configuration and demonstrate reduced apposition following treatment with a laser peripheral iridotomy.

Angle-Closure Glaucoma

Angle-closure glaucoma can present clinically with elevated IOP, pain, redness, blurry vision, and a mid-dilated pupil. Gonioscopy is essential in the diagnosis of angle closure. However, corneal edema may preclude visualization of the iridocorneal angle during an acute angle closure episode. Ultrasound can be helpful to document appositional angle closure and to identify the causes of secondary angle-closure glaucoma (discussed below). UBM is particularly useful in the diagnosis of pupillary block and demonstrating the convex iris configuration secondary to pressure differentials between the anterior and posterior chambers [7].

Dark room provocative testing may also be combined with UBM to demonstrate spontaneous occlusion of the angle under decreased illumination [8]. Determining an occludable angle can be difficult since it is dependent on operator experience as inadvertent indentation with the UBM may artificially widen the angle.

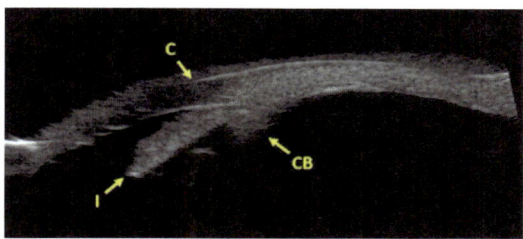

Fig. 6.2 Ultrasound biomicroscopy image of the irido-corneal angle in a patient with plateau iris syndrome demonstrating an anteriorly positioned ciliary process behind the peripheral iris. The cornea (C), iris (I), and ciliary body (CB) are marked

Plateau Iris Syndrome

Anteriorly positioned ciliary processes in plateau iris syndrome result in an atypical iris configuration, where anterior rotation of the peripheral iris leads to acute or chronic primary angle closure. This anatomical variation also prevents iridotomy from improving the angle configuration. UBM can confirm a plateau iris configuration by demonstrating the presence of a "double-hump" sign and anteriorly positioned ciliary processes (Fig. 6.2) [9].

Lens-Induced Angle Closure

Abnormalities of the lens may cause secondary glaucoma and limit thorough evaluation due to media opacities or corneal edema. Ultrasound overcomes the limitations of poor visualization to exclude other causes of glaucoma and properly address the underlying pathology. Phacolytic glaucoma resulting from a hypermature cataract can result in elevated IOP and inflammation. In cases where anterior chamber opacification occurs, ultrasound can demonstrate the characteristic findings of a morgagnian cataract: liquefied cortical material, an inferiorly displaced nucleus and thinner than normal lens. A large, cataractous lens may also cause angle closure in which ultrasound can detect lens thickening, a shallow anterior chamber, and indications of pupillary block. Ultrasound in acute angle closure secondary to

lens dislocation would demonstrate anterior lens displacement and, as important, rule out posterior segment abnormalities.

Intraocular Tumors

Ocular tumors may cause glaucoma by different mechanisms depending on the location in the anterior or posterior segment. Anterior segment tumors such as iris nevi, melanocytomas, benign adenomas, uveal melanomas, and metastases may directly invade the anterior chamber angle to affect outflow pathways or secondarily cause angle closure. Posterior segment tumors such as large choroidal melanomas and metastatic tumors in the choroid can displace the lens anteriorly to cause angle narrowing. Ultrasound can aid in differentiating between cystic and solid lesions in addition to permitting visualization of lesions behind the iris.

Intraocular Hemorrhages

Intraocular hemorrhages not only obscure visualization but may also cause glaucoma. In the setting of an anterior chamber hyphema, vitreous hemorrhage, subvitreal hemorrhage, or subretinal and subchoroidal hemorrhage, degenerated red blood cells or macrophages that have phagocytized hemoglobin may obstruct the trabecular meshwork to elevate IOP or posterior chamber forces may cause forward displacement of the vitreous and lens-iris diaphragm to shallow the anterior chamber and impede outflow. Ultrasound can be useful to visualize the anterior and posterior chamber and demonstrate diffuse vitreous opacities, dense subvitreal hemorrhage, or solid subretinal clots.

Choroidal Effusions

Choroidal effusions can occur from spontaneous uveal effusion syndrome, hypotony, reactions to systemic medications such as topiramate, a thickened sclera that obstructs outflow in

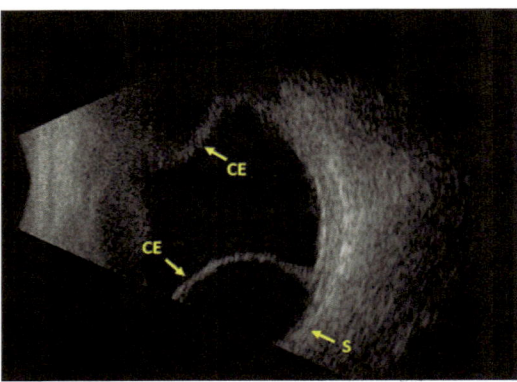

Fig. 6.3 Transverse B-scan image demonstrating large peripheral choroidal effusions in an eye with an overfiltering tube shunt device and low intraocular pressure in the postoperative period following glaucoma surgery. The choroidal effusions (CE) and sclera (S) are marked

nanophthalmos, or elevated episcleral venous pressure secondary to arteriovenous malformations or thyroid orbitopathy [10]. Choroidal effusions can cause forward rotation of the lens-iris diaphragm, resulting in increased myopia, anterior chamber shallowing, and secondary angle closure [11]. Ultrasound of the posterior chamber can show peripheral ciliochoroidal detachments (Fig. 6.3). In subtle cases, UBM may be more sensitive than conventional ultrasound in detecting shallow anterior effusions.

Inflammatory Diseases

Intraocular inflammation has the potential to cause glaucoma through various mechanisms depending on the anterior or posterior location of the uveitis. Anterior uveitis can cause elevated IOP by disrupting outflow pathways on the cellular level as inflammatory cells obstruct the trabecular meshwork and on the anatomical level from posterior synechiae at the pupillary margin or peripheral anterior synechiae between the iris and the cornea. UBM can demonstrate iris bombe or synechial angle closure when visualization is poor during acute inflammatory episodes. In uveitis-glaucoma-hyphema (UGH) syndrome, a malpositioned intraocular lens (IOL) mechanically chafes the iris, releasing pigment into the

anterior chamber and causing elevated IOP. UBM can aid in the diagnosis of UGH syndrome by identifying haptics of a single-piece IOL positioned in the sulcus or anterior vaulting of the IOL despite placement within the capsular bag [12]. Posterior uveitis may compromise the blood-retina barrier and result in choroidal effusion or thickening, as in Vogt-Koyanagi-Harada syndrome or sympathetic ophthalmia. The consequent anterior rotation of the lens-iris diaphragm narrows the anterior chamber and may lead to secondary angle-closure glaucoma. Ultrasound can demonstrate choroidal thickening and effusions, aiding in diagnosis and management.

Glaucoma Surgery Complications

The IOP fluctuation, low pressure, and anatomical changes associated with glaucoma surgery present a unique set of postoperative issues. Ultrasound may be useful for the evaluation and management of these complications.

Significant reductions in IOP and hypotony are risk factors for suprachoroidal hemorrhages and ciliochoroidal effusions. Malignant glaucoma is thought to occur due to the posterior misdirection of aqueous into the vitreous cavity. These entities may present with a shallow anterior chamber and high-or-normal intraocular pressure. While clinical history and examination findings can be helpful in differentiating these diagnoses, ultrasound is necessary to definitively show the serous component of choroidal effusions, low-to-medium reflectivity from blood or cellular debris following a choroidal hemorrhage, or the absence of choroidal and ciliary pathology in malignant glaucoma.

In cases of choroidal effusions or suprachoroidal hemorrhages that are managed conservatively, ultrasound may be used to monitor for resolution. If surgical intervention is being considered for a suprachoroidal hemorrhage, ultrasound can identify the blood clot undergoing lysis and aid in determining the surgical window.

A cyclodialysis cleft, in which the ciliary body separates from the scleral spur, may be a

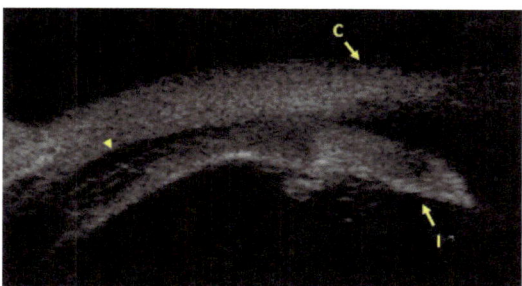

Fig. 6.4 Ultrasound biomicroscopy image of the irido-corneal angle demonstrating a small cyclodialysis cleft and fluid in the supraciliary space following trauma (yellow arrowhead). The cornea (C) and iris (I) are marked

complication following glaucoma surgery or occur after trauma. Increased uveoscleral outflow through the cleft can result in low IOP and hypotony. Repair is indicated when the cleft fails to spontaneously close and compromised vision persists. A cleft may be difficult to locate by gonioscopy secondary to size or anatomical changes. UBM can be more sensitive in locating a cleft and guiding surgical repair approaches (Fig. 6.4) [13].

Ultrasound is especially important in the management of endophthalmitis, which occurs at a higher incidence in patients who have undergone trabeculectomy surgery. Blebitis presents with inflammation of the filtering bleb and mild extension into the anterior chamber while endophthalmitis includes extension of the infection and inflammation into the posterior segment. Blebitis may be managed conservatively. In contrast, endophthalmitis requires earlier and aggressive intervention to preserve vision [14, 15]. Determining posterior segment involvement in the inflamed eye may be challenging. Ultrasound assists in determining this critical element and facilitating timely delivery of treatment.

Future Direction: Ultrasound and Optical Methods in Glaucoma

Research shows glaucomatous vision loss is due to damage to the retinal ganglion cell axons within the lamina cribrosa (LC) of the optic nerve head (ONH). Recent studies further support the

explanation by revealing significant microarchitecture changes within the LC at the early onset of experimental glaucoma [16]. Since the vision loss is irreversible in most instances, early detection is crucial for disease management. Recent studies [16–22] have suggested tissue biomechanics may determine the ONH resistance to intraocular pressure (IOP), an important risk factor for glaucomatous optic neuropathy. Moreover, several ex vivo animal studies have revealed the mechanical properties of the ONH tissue are variable across different stages of glaucoma [23, 24] and across other risk factors such as age [25–27] and race [28]. Biomechanical characteristics of ONH tissues may determine their robustness against the IOP-induced force and deformation and, particularly, the glaucomatous-related deformation on the LC as well as the peripapillary sclera (ppSC) surrounding it [17, 18, 20, 29–31]. While ex vivo studies allow for immediate access to the optic nerve head tissues, the tissue extraction and manipulation procedures both compromise the measurement accuracy. It is also clinically infeasible to investigate ocular tissue using ex vivo methods.

Over the past several years, advances in ultrasound elastography has enabled mapping of the mechanical properties of soft tissues in vivo, where elasticity is generated by analyzing the elastic behavior of tissue detected by ultrasound. Ultrasound static and shear wave elastography were successfully utilized to evaluate the elasticity of ocular tissue and differentiate glaucomatous eyes from healthy ones using several metrics [32–34]. However, the spatial resolution of ultrasound detection, which typically ranges in hundreds of microns, is insufficient to differentiate the LC from other ONH tissues. Since optical coherence tomography (OCT) has the capability to visualize ocular tissue with micrometer resolution, it could be a better candidate than ultrasound to detect the early indicator of glaucoma [21, 35–37]. Additionally, phase resolved Doppler optical coherence tomography (PRD-OCT), the functional extension of OCT, provides ultrasensitive displacement detection and allows for elasticity imaging under a minute excitation force [38–45]. In fact, PRD-OCT enabled elastography technique and optical coherence elastography (OCE) have facilitated various studies in ophthalmic applications, especially in the mechanical imaging of the anterior segment [38, 40, 46–50]. However, none of these techniques demonstrated substantial capability to assess the posterior eye segment in vivo. Y. Qu and Y. He et al. recently developed a confocal acoustic radiation force optical coherence elastography (ARF-OCE) technique to noninvasively probe the mechanical contrast of the posterior eye in vivo and provide a potential tool to study the elasticity of in vivo ONH complex [51, 52].

Static Ultrasound Elastography

The theory of static elastography (SE) relies on the fact that a compressional force deforms soft tissues to a greater extent than stiff ones. In ultrasound SE, either free hand pressure or a mechanical actuator is utilized as the source of excitation, while 2D or 3D tissue displacement is detected by ultrasonic imaging and used as a qualitative indicator of stiffness [53–55]. In prior studies, ultrasound SE demonstrates whole eye imaging, which allows for simultaneous analysis of several tissue components under the influence of different diseases [33, 34, 56, 57]. K. Agladioglu et al. performed free hand ultrasonic elastography on patients with and without primary open angle glaucoma (POAG) in vivo [33]. They compared the stiffness difference in the ocular structures between healthy and glaucomatous patients and concluded that there was a significant difference in the vitreous elasticity, with the strain ratio of the anterior and the posterior vitreous being higher for the glaucoma group.

Shear Wave Ultrasound Elastography

Dynamic elastography using the shear wave propagation velocity has also been integrated into commercially available ultrasound systems. Ultrasound shear wave elastography (SWE) uses a focused acoustic radiation force beam to deliver shear wave on the tissue, allowing for direct sub-

micron perturbation on a small region of interest (ROI) [32]. The ROI is carefully chosen to avoid invoking interactions between different biological components. Eventually, the Young's modulus or quantitative elasticity/stiffness can be mapped out using the shear wave equation that defines a linear relationship between Young's modulus and the square of shear wave speed [58]. Ultrasound SWE has been used by A. S. Dikici et al. to study the biomechanical properties of glaucomatous ONH and surrounding tissues in vivo [32]. Twenty-one consecutive primary open angle glaucoma patients and 21 healthy volunteers participated in the clinical study, which found the mean Young's modulus values of both the optic nerve and peripapillary sclera in glaucomatous eyes are significantly higher, indicating increased stiffness when compared to healthy patients [32].

Confocal Acoustic Radiation Force Optical Coherence Elastography

The confocal acoustic radiation force optical coherence elastography (ARF-OCE) technique excites and detects the elastic behavior of tissue using ultrasound and phase resolved Doppler optical coherence tomography (PRD-OCT), respectively [51, 52]. To be specific, the optical detection beam sits in parallel with the ultrasound excitation, through the aperture of a ring-shaped transducer on the same side, to ensure easy access to the posterior eye, maximum detection sensitivity based on the PRD-OCT theory. This technology allows for the quantitative assessment of tissue biomechanics through both shear wave and compressional wave analyses. Compressional wave ARF-OCE allows for real-time qualitative elasticity imaging but requires phantom calibration for quantitative results. Figure 6.5 shows the elastography generated by inducing, detecting, and analyzing the compressional wave propagating in an in vivo rabbit retina. An 8-week light treatment was performed to induce damage within the posterior eye segment, and elastography images were taken before and after at the same central retina region. Histological analyses in

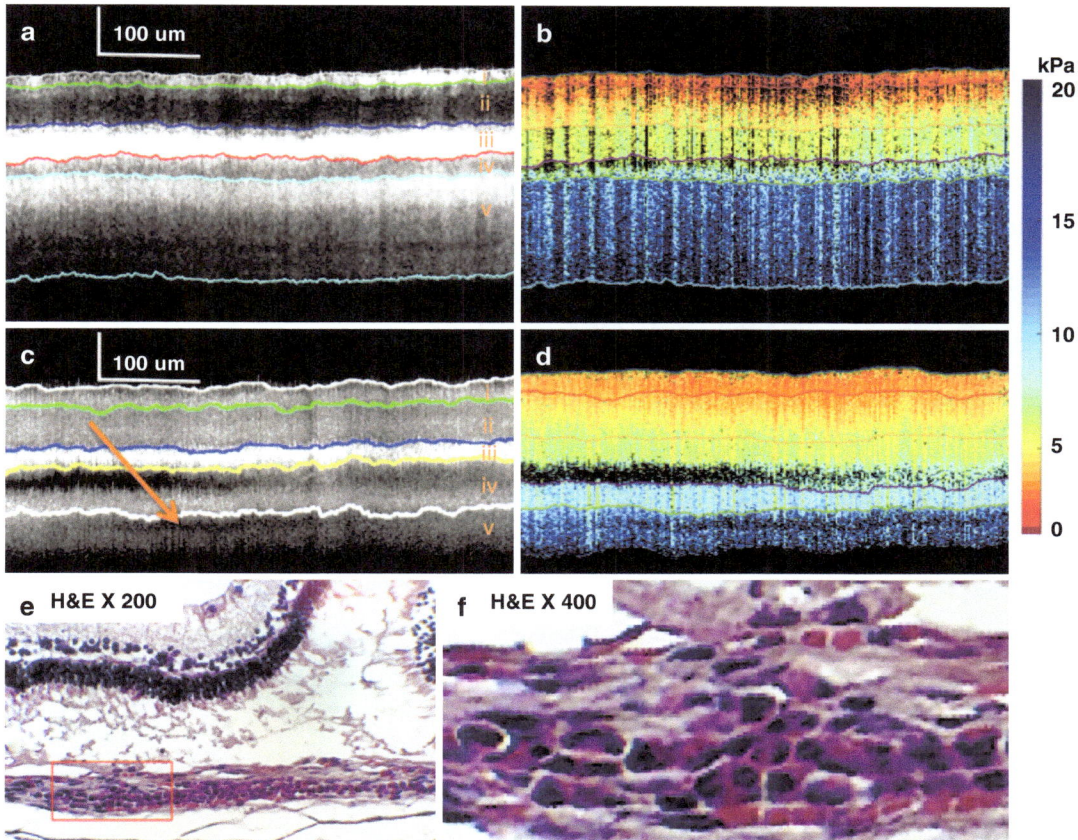

Fig. 6.5 Results obtained from in vivo rabbit retina before and after blue light treatment. (**a, b**) OCT and elastography of healthy retina. (**c, d**) OCT and elastography of retina after treatment. (**e**) H&E stain histology of light-treated retina, tissue damage, and lymphocyte infil-tration were discovered and matched to the low signal region pointed out by the orange arrow in (**c**). (**f**) Zoomed in view of histological analysis result in Fig. 6.5e (Copyright © 2018: The Authors [52])

Fig. 6.5e, f validate the treatment outcome by showing the abnormal region with inflammation in the red box. The region of inflammation might have invoked lymphocytic infiltration, which corresponds to less OCT scattering and lower stiffness compared to the surrounding choroidal tissue [59–62]. Figure 6.5c shows the corresponding OCT image, where the orange arrow points to the low signal site, which is suspected to be the inflammatory region. Mechanical contrast of the imaging area is shown by Figs. 6.5b, d and 6.6.

The confocal ARF-OCE system is also capable of quantitative elastography imaging by measuring the shear wave propagation [51, 52]. Although shear wave analysis needs more computations than compressional wave, it does not rely on phantom calibrations and may provide more precise elasticity measurements than the shear wave elastography (SWE). Several phantom studies have verified the feasibility of SWE using ARF and OCT [40, 44]. Although ex vivo mapping of the posterior ocular elasticity was reported, the technique places the ARF excitation on the opposite side of the OCT detection, which limits its application to ex vivo only since ARF cannot penetrate through the thickness of the skull and tissues behind the eye globe [63].

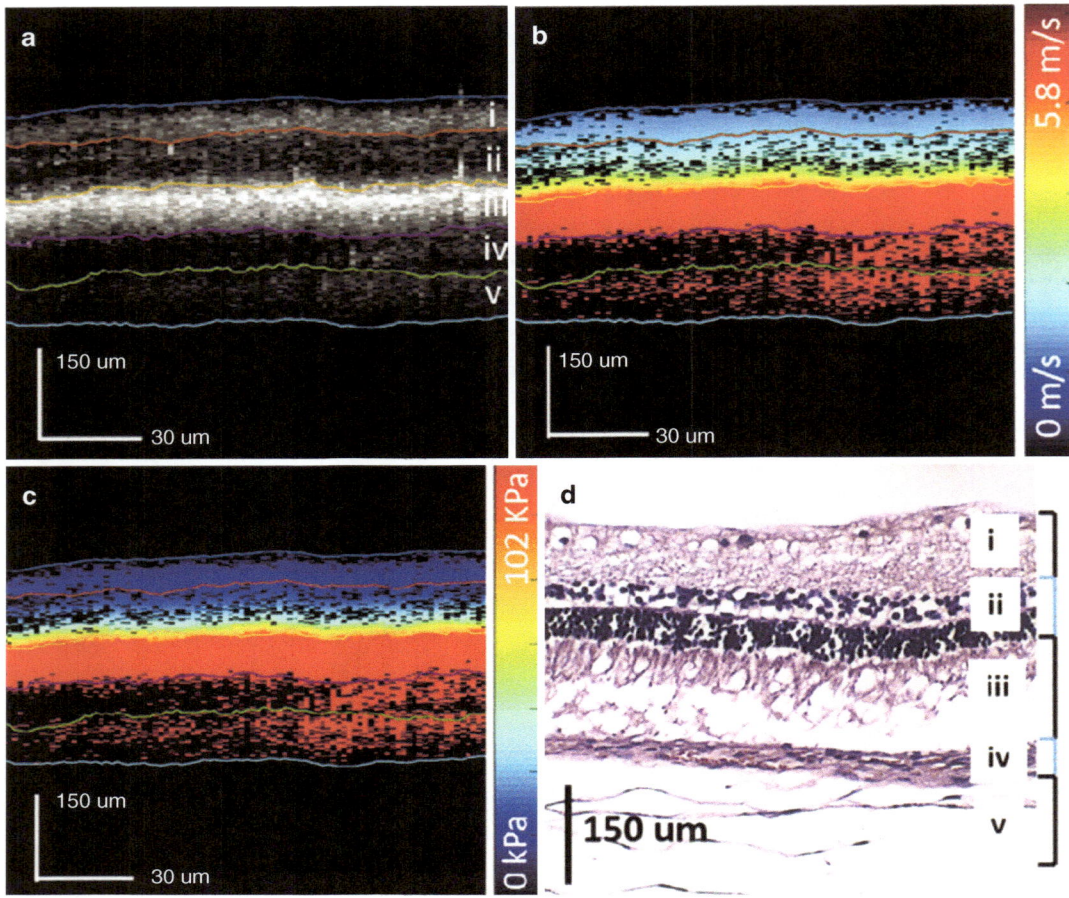

Fig. 6.6 Results of in vivo rabbit retina using shear wave ARF-OCE. (**a**) OCT cross-section. (**b**) Shear velocity map. (**c**) Elastography showing Young's modulus mapping. (**d**) H&E stain histology. (Copyright © 2019: IEEE [51])

Summary and Future Directions

Biomechanical characteristics of ocular tissues, especially the lamina cribrosa and peripapillary sclera within the optic nerve head (ONH) complex, have been hypothesized to be the earliest indicators for the development of glaucoma. From ultrasound elastography to acoustic radiation force optical coherence elastography (ARF-OCE), ultrasound has proven to be a powerful tool in the diagnosis of posterior ocular diseases. Recently, the confocal ARF-OCE technique has proven its potential in visualizing the mechanical contrast of the posterior eye. Although limitations still exist, these studies open up the possibility of studying the biomechanics of glaucoma in vivo. In further studies, it is crucial to increase the accuracy of these techniques, possibly by adopting a numerical model of the ONH, which has been well studied in the past decade [64–67], to solve for the spatial elasticity with the inverse elastography technique [68, 69]. Therefore, future study should focus on the simulation and validation of the confocal ARF-OCE technique with varies computational methods.

Acknowledgment This work was supported in part by the National Institutes of Health under Grant R01HL-125084, Grant R01HL-127271, Grant R01EY-026091, Grant R01EY-021529, Grant P41EB-015890, Grant F31EY027666, and Grant R01EY-028662 and in part by the Air Force Office of Scientific Research under Grant FA9550-14-1-0034.

Compliance with Ethical Requirements Jiun L. Do, MD, PhD, Youmin He, Yueqiao Qu, PhD, and Qifa Zhou, PhD, declare they have no conflict of interest. Zhongping Chen, PhD, has a financial interest in OCT Medical Imaging, Inc., which did not support this work, so there is no conflict of interest. No human studies were carried out by the authors for this chapter. All rabbit experiments were performed with adherence to the guidelines set forth by the University of California, Irvine Institutional Animal Care and Use Committee (IACUC).

References

1. Pavlin CJ, Foster FS. Ultrasound biomicroscopy. High-frequency ultrasound imaging of the eye at microscopic resolution. Radiol Clin N Am. 1998;36:1047–58.
2. Darnley-Fisch DA, Byrne SF, Hughes JR, Parrish RK, Feuer WJ. Contact B-scan echography in the assessment of optic nerve cupping. Am J Ophthalmol. 1990;109:55–61.
3. Thau A, et al. New classification system for pediatric glaucoma: implications for clinical care and a research registry. Curr Opin Ophthalmol. 2018;29:385–94.
4. Sampaolesi R, Caruso R. Ocular echometry in the diagnosis of congenital glaucoma. Arch Ophthalmol. 1982;100:574–7.
5. Gupta V, Jha R, Srinivasan G, Dada T, Sihota R. Ultrasound biomicroscopic characteristics of the anterior segment in primary congenital glaucoma. J Am Assoc Pediatr Ophthalmol Strabismus. 2007;11:546–50.
6. Potash SD, Tello C, Liebmann J, Ritch R. Ultrasound biomicroscopy in pigment dispersion syndrome. Ophthalmology. 1994;101:332–9.
7. Aslanides IM, et al. High frequency ultrasound imaging in pupillary block glaucoma. Br J Ophthalmol. 1995;79:972–6.
8. Smith SD, et al. Evaluation of the anterior chamber angle in glaucoma: a report by the American Academy of Ophthalmology. Ophthalmology. 2013;120:1985–97.
9. Pavlin CJ, Ritch R, Foster FS. Ultrasound biomicroscopy in plateau iris syndrome. Am J Ophthalmol. 1992;113:390–5.
10. Man X, Costa R, Ayres BM, Moroi SE. Acetazolamide-induced bilateral ciliochoroidal effusion syndrome in plateau iris configuration. Am J Ophthalmol Case Rep. 2016;3:14–7.
11. Fourman S. Angle-closure glaucoma complicating ciliochoroidal detachment. Ophthalmology. 1989;96:646–53.
12. Piette S, et al. Ultrasound biomicroscopy in uveitis-glaucoma-hyphema syndrome. Am J Ophthalmol. 2002;133:839–41.
13. Gentile RC, et al. Diagnosis of traumatic cyclodialysis by ultrasound biomicroscopy. Ophthalmic Surg Lasers. 1996;27:97–105.
14. Ciulla TA, Beck AD, Topping TM, Baker AS. Blebitis, early endophthalmitis, and late endophthalmitis after glaucoma-filtering surgery. Ophthalmology. 1997;104:986–95.
15. Ayyala RS, Bellows AR, Thomas JV, Hutchinson BT. Bleb infections: clinically different courses of "blebitis" and endophthalmitis. Ophthalmic Surg Lasers. 1997;28:452–60.
16. Burgoyne CF, Downs JC. Premise and prediction–how optic nerve head biomechanics underlies the susceptibility and clinical behavior of the aged optic nerve head. J Glaucoma. 2008;17(4):318.
17. Nguyen TD, Ethier CR. Biomechanical assessment in models of glaucomatous optic neuropathy. Exp Eye Res. 2015;141:125–38.
18. Sigal IA, Ethier CR. Biomechanics of the optic nerve head. Exp Eye Res. 2009;88(4):799–807.
19. Burgoyne CF, et al. The optic nerve head as a biomechanical structure: a new paradigm for understanding the role of IOP-related stress and strain in the pathophysiology of glaucomatous optic nerve head damage. Prog Retin Eye Res. 2005;24(1):39–73.
20. Sigal IA, et al. Factors influencing optic nerve head biomechanics. Invest Ophthalmol Vis Sci. 2005;46(11):4189–99.
21. Sigal IA, et al. A method to estimate biomechanics and mechanical properties of optic nerve head tissues from parameters measurable using optical coherence tomography. IEEE Trans Med Imaging. 2014;33(6):1381–9.
22. Coudrillier B, et al. Biomechanics of the human posterior sclera: age-and glaucoma-related changes measured using inflation testing. Invest Ophthalmol Vis Sci. 2012;53(4):1714–28.
23. Girard MJ, et al. Biomechanical changes in the sclera of monkey eyes exposed to chronic IOP elevations. Invest Ophthalmol Vis Sci. 2011;52(8):5656–69.
24. Grytz R, et al. Material properties of the posterior human sclera. J Mech Behav Biomed Mater. 2014;29:602–17.
25. Quigley HA, Broman AT. The number of people with glaucoma worldwide in 2010 and 2020. Br J Ophthalmol. 2006;90(3):262–7.
26. Fazio MA, et al. Age-related changes in human peripapillary scleral strain. Biomech Model Mechanobiol. 2014;13(3):551–63.
27. Grytz R, et al. Age-and race-related differences in human scleral material properties. Invest Ophthalmol Vis Sci. 2014;55(12):8163–72.
28. Fazio MA, et al. Human scleral structural stiffness increases more rapidly with age in donors of African descent compared to donors of European descent. Invest Ophthalmol Vis Sci. 2014;55(11):7189–98.
29. Ethier CR, Johnson M, Ruberti J. Ocular biomechanics and biotransport. Annu Rev Biomed Eng. 2004;6:249–73.
30. Girard MJ, et al. In vivo optic nerve head biomechanics: performance testing of a three-dimensional tracking algorithm. J R Soc Interface. 2013;10(87):20130459.

31. Woo SL, et al. Mathematical model of the corneo-scleral shell as applied to intraocular pressure-volume relations and applanation tonometry. Ann Biomed Eng. 1972;1(1):87–98.

32. Dikici AS, et al. In vivo evaluation of the biomechanical properties of optic nerve and peripapillary structures by ultrasonic shear wave elastography in glaucoma. Iran J Radiol. 2016;13(2):e36849.

33. Agladioglu K, et al. An evaluation of ocular elasticity using real-time ultrasound elastography in primary open-angle glaucoma. Br J Radiol. 2016;89(1060):20150429.

34. Özen Ö, et al. Evaluation of the optic nerve and scleral-choroidal-retinal layer with ultrasound elastography in glaucoma and physiological optic nerve head cupping. Med Ultrason. 2018;20(1):76–9.

35. Wang S, Larin KV. Optical coherence elastography for tissue characterization: a review. J Biophotonics. 2015;8(4):279–302.

36. Kennedy BF, Kennedy KM, Sampson DD. A review of optical coherence elastography: fundamentals, techniques and prospects. IEEE J Sel Top Quantum Electron. 2014;20(2):272–88.

37. Devalla SK, et al. A deep learning approach to digitally stain optical coherence tomography images of the optic nerve head. Invest Ophthalmol Vis Sci. 2018;59(1):63–74.

38. Qu Y, et al. Quantified elasticity mapping of retinal layers using synchronized acoustic radiation force optical coherence elastography. Biomed Opt Express. 2018;9(9):4054–63.

39. Qu Y, et al. Miniature probe for mechanical properties of vascular lesions using acoustic radiation force optical coherence elastography (Conference Presentation). In: Optical elastography and tissue biomechanics III. International Society for Optics and Photonics; 2016.

40. Zhu J, et al. 3D mapping of elastic modulus using shear wave optical micro-elastography. Sci Rep. 2016;6:35499.

41. Zhu J, et al. Longitudinal shear wave imaging for elasticity mapping using optical coherence elastography. Appl Phys Lett. 2017;110(20):201101.

42. Zhu J, et al. Imaging shear wave propagation for elastic measurement using OCT Doppler variance method. In: Optical coherence tomography and coherence domain optical methods in biomedicine XX. International Society for Optics and Photonics; 2016.

43. Qu Y, et al. Acoustic radiation force optical coherence elastography of corneal tissue. IEEE J Sel Top Quantum Electron. 2016;22(3):288–94.

44. Zhu J, et al. Imaging and characterizing shear wave and shear modulus under orthogonal acoustic radiation force excitation using OCT Doppler variance method. Opt Lett. 2015;40(9):2099–102.

45. Zhu J, et al. Coaxial excitation longitudinal shear wave measurement for quantitative elasticity assessment using phase-resolved optical coherence elastography. Opt Lett. 2018;43(10):2388–91.

46. Li J, et al. Air-pulse OCE for assessment of age-related changes in mouse cornea in vivo. Laser Phys Lett. 2014;11(6):065601.

47. Li J, et al. Dynamic optical coherence tomography measurements of elastic wave propagation in tissue-mimicking phantoms and mouse cornea in vivo. J Biomed Opt. 2013;18(12):121503.

48. Han Z, et al. Optical coherence elastography assessment of corneal viscoelasticity with a modified Rayleigh-Lamb wave model. J Mech Behav Biomed Mater. 2017;66:87–94.

49. Roy AS, et al. Air-puff associated quantification of non-linear biomechanical properties of the human cornea in vivo. J Mech Behav Biomed Mater. 2015;48:173–82.

50. Ambroziński Ł, et al. Acoustic micro-tapping for non-contact 4D imaging of tissue elasticity. Sci Rep. 2016;6:38967.

51. He Y, et al. Confocal shear wave acoustic radiation force optical coherence elastography for imaging and quantification of the in vivo posterior eye. IEEE J Sel Top Quantum Electron. 2019;25(1):1–7.

52. Qu Y, et al. In vivo elasticity mapping of posterior ocular layers using acoustic radiation force optical coherence elastography. Invest Ophthalmol Vis Sci. 2018;59(1):455–61.

53. Varghese T. Quasi-static ultrasound elastography. Ultrasound Clin. 2009;4(3):323.

54. Treece G, et al. Real-time quasi-static ultrasound elastography. Interface Focus. 2011;1(4):540–52.

55. Papadacci C, Bunting EA, Konofagou EE. 3D quasi-static ultrasound elastography with plane wave in vivo. IEEE Trans Med Imaging. 2017;36(2):357–65.

56. Vural M, et al. The evaluation of the retrobulbar orbital fat tissue and optic nerve with strain ratio elastography. Med Ultrason. 2015;17(1):45–8.

57. İnal M, et al. Evaluation of the optic nerve using strain and shear wave elastography in patients with multiple sclerosis and healthy subjects. Med Ultrason. 2017;19(1):39–44.

58. Li G-Y, Cao Y. Mechanics of ultrasound elastography. Proc Math Phys Eng Sci. 2017;473(2199):20160841.

59. Liu L, et al. Imaging the subcellular structure of human coronary atherosclerosis using micro–optical coherence tomography. Nat Med. 2011;17(8):1010.

60. Bufi N, et al. Human primary immune cells exhibit distinct mechanical properties that are modified by inflammation. Biophys J. 2015;108(9):2181–90.

61. Cai X, et al. Connection between biomechanics and cytoskeleton structure of lymphocyte and Jurkat cells: an AFM study. Micron. 2010;41(3):257–62.

62. Liang X, et al. Optical micro-scale mapping of dynamic biomechanical tissue properties. Opt Express. 2008;16(15):11052–65.

63. Song S, et al. Quantitative shear-wave optical coherence elastography with a programmable phased array ultrasound as the wave source. Opt Lett. 2015;40(21):5007–10.

64. Sigal IA, et al. Reconstruction of human optic nerve heads for finite element modeling. Technol Health Care. 2005;13(4):313–29.

65. Grytz R, et al. Lamina cribrosa thickening in early glaucoma predicted by a microstructure motivated growth and remodeling approach. Mech Mater. 2012;44:99–109.

66. Sigal IA, et al. Modeling individual-specific human optic nerve head biomechanics. Part II: influence of material properties. Biomech Model Mechanobiol. 2009;8(2):99–109.

67. Roberts MD, et al. Correlation between local stress and strain and lamina cribrosa connective tissue volume fraction in normal monkey eyes. Invest Ophthalmol Vis Sci. 2010;51(1):295–307.

68. Govindjee S, Mihalic PA. Computational methods for inverse finite elastostatics. Comput Methods Appl Mech Eng. 1996;136(1–2):47–57.

69. Lu J, Zhou X, Raghavan ML. Inverse elastostatic stress analysis in pre-deformed biological structures: demonstration using abdominal aortic aneurysms. J Biomech. 2007;40(3):693–6.

Imaging Aqueous Outflow

7

Ralitsa T. Loewen, Susannah Waxman,
Hirut Kollech, Jonathan Vande Geest,
and Nils A. Loewen

Introduction

The flow of aqueous humor is difficult to study due to its low rate of production, about 2.5 ± 1.0 μL (mean $\pm$ SD) per minute [1] and its slow rate of drainage. The minuscule size of the outflow pathways and vessels and the variable characteristics of their contents (aqueous, blood, or lymphatic) present an additional challenge. The cause of increased intraocular pressure (IOP) in primary open angle glaucoma (POAG) was long thought to be secondary to increased outflow resistance of the trabecular meshwork (TM), which limits aqueous outflow from the eye [2, 3]. However, research [4–8] and data from clini-cal TM ablation in thousands of patients [9–12] show it fails to lower IOP to the pressure level in the recipient episcleral veins, strongly suggesting that over half of resistance resides in the distal outflow tract, downstream of the TM and Schlemm's canal (SC). An additional deep ablation of valve-like structures at collector channel orifices located in the outer SC wall fails to lower IOP further [13–15]. The loci and substrates of distal outflow resistance are unknown, but critical to identify. To overcome these barriers and permit effective clinical IOP reduction, research has been directed at identifying the mechanism and anatomic locus of post-TM outflow resistance and test two hypotheses: (1) distal outflow resistance resides in the collector channels (CC), intrascleral plexus (ISP), or aqueous veins (AV); (2) this resistance can be overcome by treatment with vasodilatory and vasculogenic agents.

In this chapter, we will focus on the conventional outflow system but also mention techniques used to visualize uveoscleral, including uveolymphatic, outflow. A brief, non-exhaustive review of experiments and discoveries in chronological order is helpful to understand the research efforts started almost 200 years ago.

R. T. Loewen
University of Pittsburgh, Department
of Ophthalmology, Pittsburgh, PA, USA

S. Waxman
University of Pittsburgh, School of Medicine,
Interdisciplinary Biomedical Graduate Program,
Pittsburgh, PA, USA

H. Kollech
Computational Modeling and Simulation Program,
Pittsburgh, PA, USA

J. Vande Geest
Department of Bioengineering, University
of Pittsburgh, Pittsburgh, PA, USA

N. A. Loewen (✉)
University of Würzburg, Department
of Ophthalmology, Würzburg, Germany

History of Qualitative Outflow Imaging

Known for his pathology studies on cadavers, when German anatomist Friedrich Schlemm

© Springer Nature Switzerland AG 2020
R. Varma et al. (eds.), *Advances in Ocular Imaging in Glaucoma*, Essentials in Ophthalmology,
https://doi.org/10.1007/978-3-030-43847-0_7

(1795–1858) first described a unique vessel encircling the cornea—now known as Schlemm's canal—in 1830 [16], interest in the role of aqueous outflow in glaucoma and the vessels associated with aqueous outflow rapidly increased. Schlemm described a "thin walled canal, which I discovered in 1827, in the eye of a man who had hung himself, so that it was filled with blood and in which one could easily insert a small bristle after cut down through the cornea and sclera." This sounds similar to the techniques of inducing episcleral venous blood reflux to identify Schlemm's canal and ab externo cut down to identify and probe Schlemm's canal, respectively.

Adjacent "suction vessels" radiating from the limbus were identified via injection of glutin glue mixed with lead oxide into the perilimbal tissue by the Polish anatomist Ludwik Karol Teichmann-Stawiarski in 1861 [17] (Fig. 7.1). Two German ophthalmologists, Gustav Schwalbe in 1870 [18] and Theodor Leber in 1873 [19], performed the first canalograms by intracamerally injecting dyes with different particle sizes to investigate Schlemm's canal. Schwalbe originally interpreted the canal as a lymphatic vessel but later debated its venous features, a remarkable insight given the mixed origin of Schlemm's canal has only recently been confirmed [20–22]. Schwalbe was convinced a direct communication of clefts existed between the anterior chamber and Schlemm's canal. French ophthalmologist André

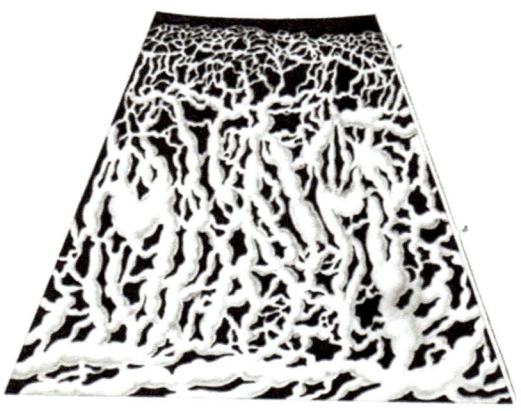

Fig. 7.1 Early depiction by Ludwik Karol Teichmann-Stawiarski of perilimbal drainage from 1861 as a "suction vessel system" [17]

Rochon-Duvigneaud (1892) disagreed [23] calling it an osmotic process. Leber [24] described Schlemm's canal as covered by a non-perforated, uninterrupted cell layer before German ophthalmologist Gustav Gutmann characterized it in 1895 as an open communication dependent on the particle size of the ink injected [25]. In the same year, Bentzen and Leber compared outflow of different dyes in normal and glaucomatous enucleated eyes and concluded: "in all cases of glaucoma examined, in simple glaucoma (acute or chronic), in angle closure and secondary glaucoma, there was a considerable reduction in filtration from the anterior chamber compared to the normal eye" [26].

After further studies, in 1903, Leber hypothesized there were connecting vessels between Schlemm's canal and the episcleral veins [27]. In 1921, Erich Seidel, a German ophthalmologist who described fluorescein dilution as an aqueous humor leak test (Seidel's test) (Seidel 1921), did extensive ex vivo and in vivo dye canalogram studies to highlight these outflow vessels and created a model of pigment-induced glaucoma in a rabbit [28]. In 1922, he determined the pressure gradient across the TM and the episcleral venous pressure [29]. By now, many substances and methods of injection had been tried. Ada Stübel, a German veterinarian and an ophthalmologist, mused in 1922 about the flurry of techniques used to trace outflow [30]: "One would inject colored water, milk, or mercury directly into the larger vessels or one would target them indirectly by tissue injection mostly with viscous glue mixtures (Teichmann) or oil-based paints (Gerota), in addition to some water-based dyes (Mascagni)." She took advantage of her knowledge of both human and animal models and applied hydrogen peroxide to tissue surfaces or injected traces of it into specimens. This induced fine bubbles ("due to catalase") in lymphatic channels that could be seen under the microscope. In both human and porcine eyes, she observed a network of fine channels with biochemical characteristics of lymphatic vessels located superficially anterior to Schlemm's canal.

American ophthalmologist Georgiana Dvorak-Theobald, MD, reconstructed anastomoses

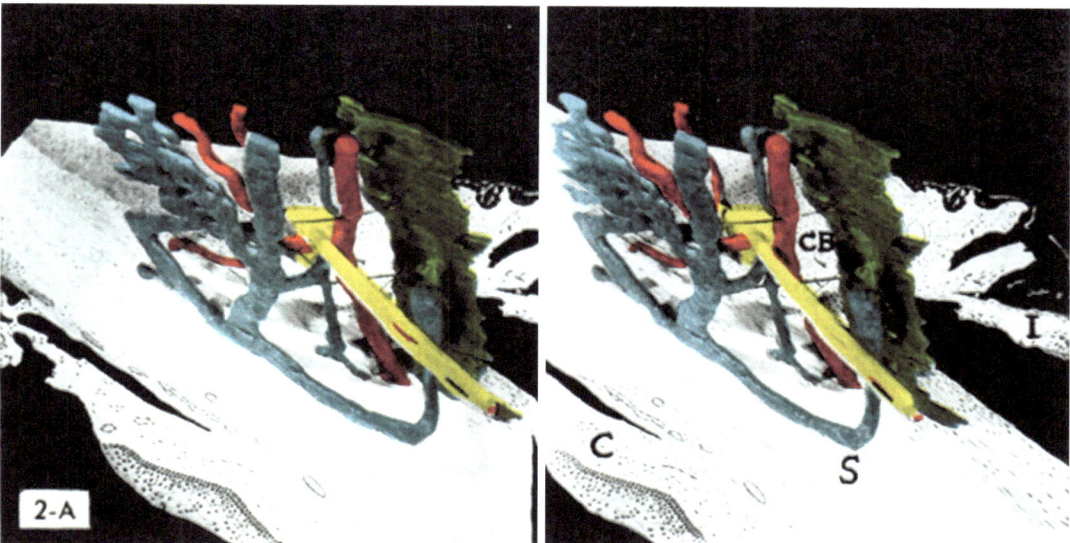

Fig. 7.2 Three-dimensional projection by Georgiana Dvorak-Theobald of paraffin sections from 1934 show the human nasal outflow tract anatomy with S, Schlemm's canal (green), episcleral veins (blue), arteries (red), and nerves (yellow). Images can be merged for a 3D impression by crossing the eyes. C, conjunctiva; I, iris; CB, cili-ary body [31]. (This figure is taken from an article, "Schlemm's Canal: Its Anastomoses and Anatomic Relations" in the Trans Am Ophthalmol Soc 1934; 32:574-595 and republished with permission of the American Ophthalmological Society)

and anatomic relations of Schlemm's canal and episcleral vessels in sophisticated three-dimensional, magnified wax projections in 1934 [31] (Fig. 7.2). In the same year, the British eye doctor, Basil Graves, provided detailed drawings of the perilimbal flow and described empty appearing vessels, later to be defined as aqueous vessels [32] (Fig. 7.3). The renowned American ocular pathologist Jonas S. Friedenwald, MD, assembled serial microscopy sections in compound drawings in 1936 [33]. British ophthalmologist of Austrian birth, Arnold Loewenstein, MD, described in 1940 vessels appearing to be empty as if filled with water and seemed to be connected to episcleral veins [34]. These vessels were examined more extensively by Czech-born American ophthalmologist Karl Wolfgang Ascher, MD, in 1942 [35]. Ascher manipulated these "aqueous veins" pharmacologically and physically by compressing confluent recipient vessel with a glass rod, a test considered negative when venous blood displaced the aqueous in a connected vessel upon compression of a common recipient vessel [35, 36]. This finding indicated impaired trabecular facility and reduced ability to displace blood in the connected venous arm of a given perilimbal vessels. Aqueous vessels were soon confirmed in 1947 by Dutch Steven De Vries [37] with further research by Swiss ophthalmologist Hans Goldmann [38] in 1948. Goldmann's research was instrumental in the understanding of aqueous veins. In 1941, he determined the volume of the anterior chamber, then 4 years later detected the aqueous veins and proved they contained aqueous in 1949. One year later, he measured aqueous production by fluorescein dilution curves and subsequently coined the formula determining outflow facility. In a series of neoprene cast studies of Schlemm's canal and aqueous veins, Norman Ashton, CBE, FRS, DSc, the first ophthalmic pathologist in the United Kingdom, reconstructed the outflow tract in 3D as plasticine and wire models, showing aqueous veins emerge directly from Schlemm's canal while others are connected to the superficial and deep scleral plexuses or their communicating

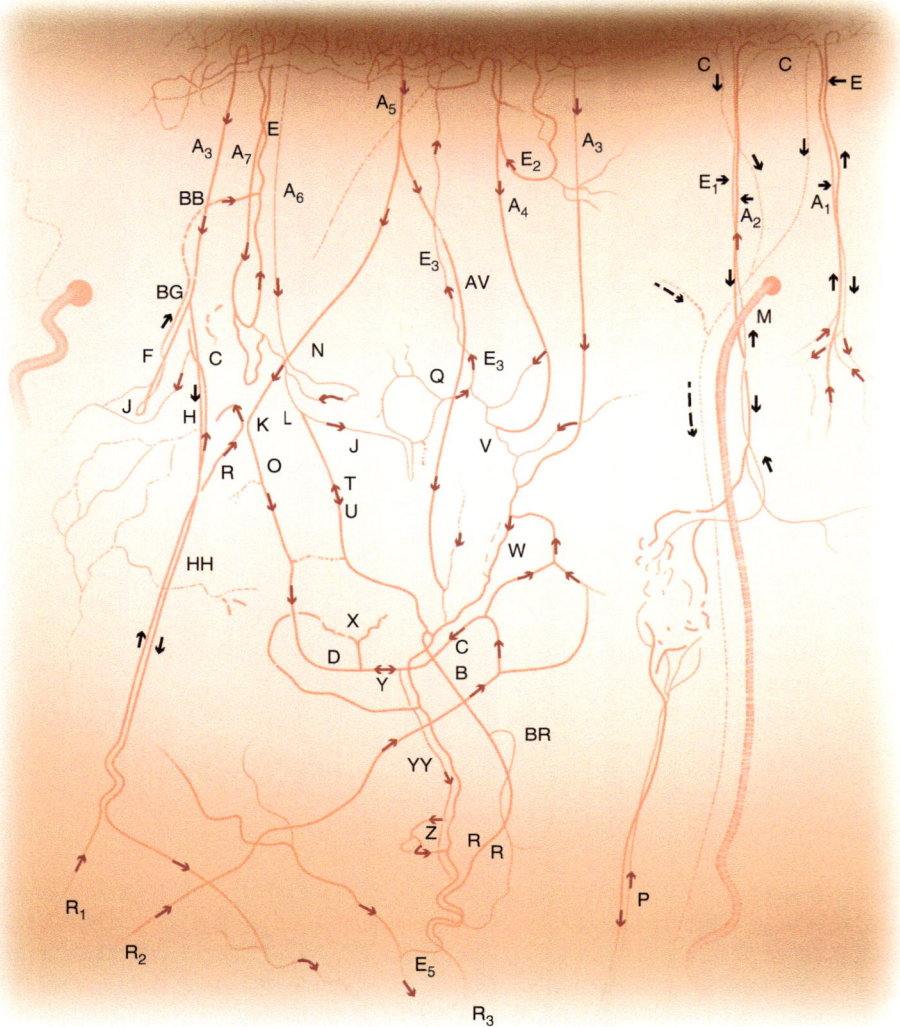

Fig. 7.3 Perilimbal flow in the human eye with flow directions by Basil Graves (1934) [32]. In later observations, empty appearing vessels were defined as aqueous vessels

branches [39] (Fig. 7.4). Loewenstein characterized the human outflow system in more detail in 1951 and provided their clinical context in enucleated eyes [40]. In 1951, D. P. Greaves and E. S. Perkins observed in a rabbit model that aqueous veins constrict after electrical stimulation of the cervical sympathetic nerves and increasing the intraocular pressure displaces more aqueous into the aqueous veins [41]. Other investigators reported outer wall changes of Schlemm's canal, obstruction of collector channel openings, and diminished or collapsing collector channels and intrascleral veins as pathologic changes in glaucoma [42–44].

According to Bruce E. Cohan [45], Italian Croci (1932) and Russian Baltin (1945 [46]) attempted to use intracameral injection of thorotrast, a suspension containing particles of radioactive and radiodense thorium dioxide with a particle size of 7–10 microns, to trace aqueous flow along what is now known as the conventional outflow system. While they failed, they detected

neoprene cast of Schlemm's canal   high power view of neoprene cast

plasticine and wire model of neoprene cast   drawing of neoprene cast

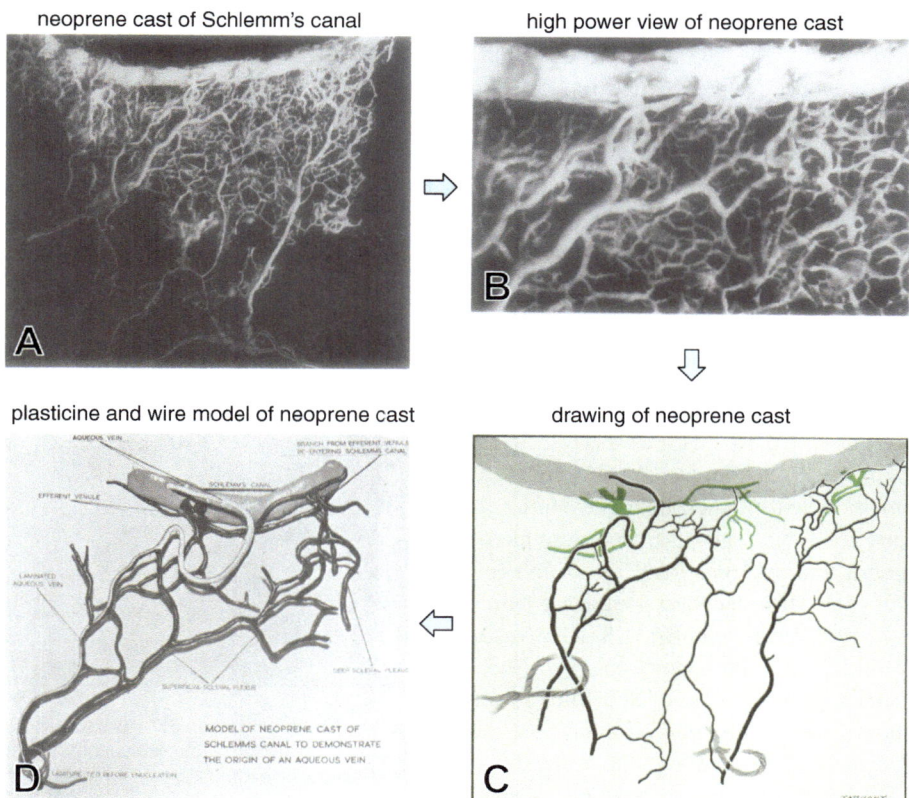

Fig. 7.4 Historic neoprene casts at different magnifications (**a, b**). Drawing (**c**) and plasticine and wire model of cast (**d**) [39]

the marker in the suprachoroidal space and iris stroma—now recognized to be part of the uveo-scleral outflow route—and often phagocytosed by histiocytes. In contrast, in 1955, Belgium J. François et al. [47] using monkey and human eyes, deployed thorium dioxide with a particle size of 0.1 micron or, alternatively, ethyl stearate with particles varying from one to four microns. They demonstrated a direct communication between the anterior chamber and Schlemm's canal through pores that limited uptake to a size below 2.4 micron. Cohan recognized the need for live imaging of outflow and echoed Stübel by reiterating the importance of avoiding artifacts caused by unbalanced nonphysiological solutions, by solvents containing particles, or by the high injection pressure needed for viscous fillers such as neoprene [45, 48]. In 1968, J. W. Rohen and F. J. Rentsch explored different outflow tract cast materials and created detailed corrosion casts of human Schlemm's canal [49], a technique

later repeated by John C. Morrison, MD, in great detail with scanning electron microscopy and methylmethacrylate in the rat [50]. Traditional histology obtained by light microscopy helped distinguish normal [51–53] from glaucomatous eyes [54–56]. Electron microscopy and molecular studies [57–59] identified various additional changes, mostly in the TM. Cheryl R. Hann, MS, observed a reduced number of collector channels in glaucomatous eyes [56]. More recently, various investigators have imaged the outflow structures at a higher resolution and greater depth with computer-supported 3D reconstruction as detailed in section "Depth-Resolved Imaging".

Depth-Resolved Imaging

As clinical evidence for post-trabecular outflow resistance became better established [60, 61], greater interest fell on post-trabecular outflow elements.

In searching for possible sites of outflow resistance downstream of the TM, the ability to distinguish distal and proximal features of the outflow tract becomes increasingly important. Advances in imaging allowed for optical sectioning and accurate 3D reconstruction of tissue. While computationally intensive, this is far less intensive and error-prone than manual sectioning and reconstruction.

It was not until 2010 that spectral domain optical coherence tomography was used to visualize conventional outflow structures ex vivo and in vivo by Larry Kagemann, PhD, et al. [62], a method subsequently improved [62–66] (Fig. 7.5). In 2011, Cheryl R. Hann et al. deployed 3D micro-computed tomography, a method with a theoretical resolution of one micron or lower and was used here at two microns and five microns voxel resolution [67] (Fig. 7.6). In 2014, Howard Hughes Medical Institute research scientist Krishnakumar Kizhatil, PhD, et al. used confocal microscopy to characterize development of Schlemm's canal from blood vessels in the mouse limbus [20], and in 2017, Jose M. Gonzalez Jr., et al. utilized two-photon microscopy in live mice to characterize contractile features of the outflow tract [68].

In subsequent studies, the complete porcine outflow tract was imaged in 3D via optical clearing and ribbon-scanning confocal microscopy with a resolution limit of 365 nm [69]. Acquiring these data sets took 1–2 days and was computationally intensive, with a computation time of

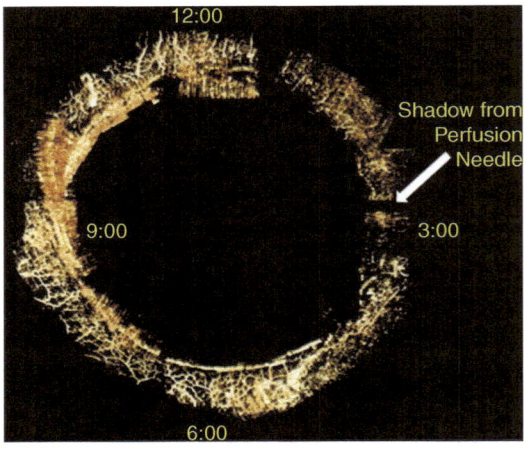

Fig. 7.5 Frontal view of 3D visualization of aqueous humor outflow structures in humans by spectral domain optical coherence tomography. S, superior (12:00), N, nasal (9:00), I, inferior (6:00), T, temporal (3:00). (Courtesy of Dr. Kagemann) [63]

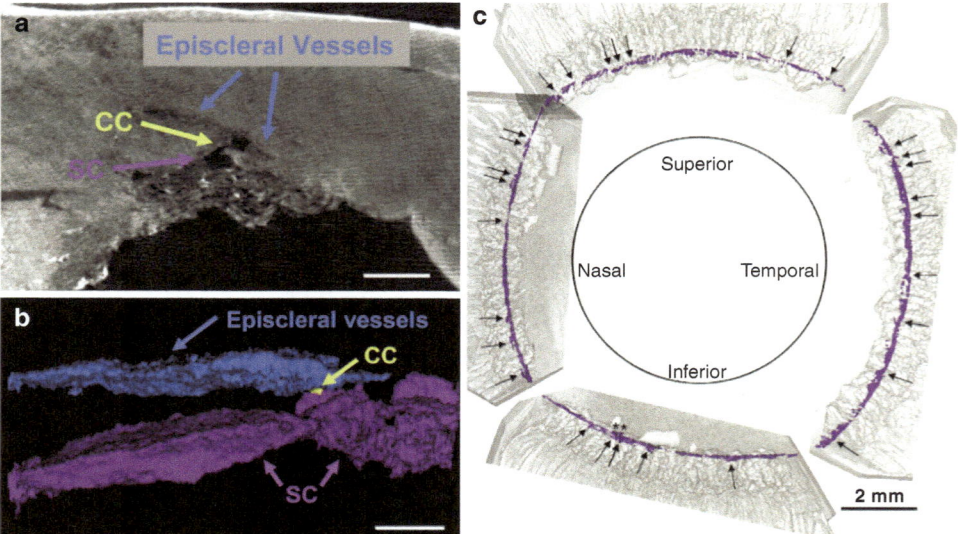

Fig. 7.6 3D micro-CT of fixed tissue can be used for examination of the trabecular meshwork, Schlemm's canal (SC), collector channels (CC), and episcleral vessel of the distal outflow pathway. Sagittal view (**a**); subtractive view of empty appearing SC, CC, and episcleral vessel (**b**); frontal view of assembled anterior segment (**c**). Black arrows = collector channels. (Courtesy of Dr. Fautsch) [67]

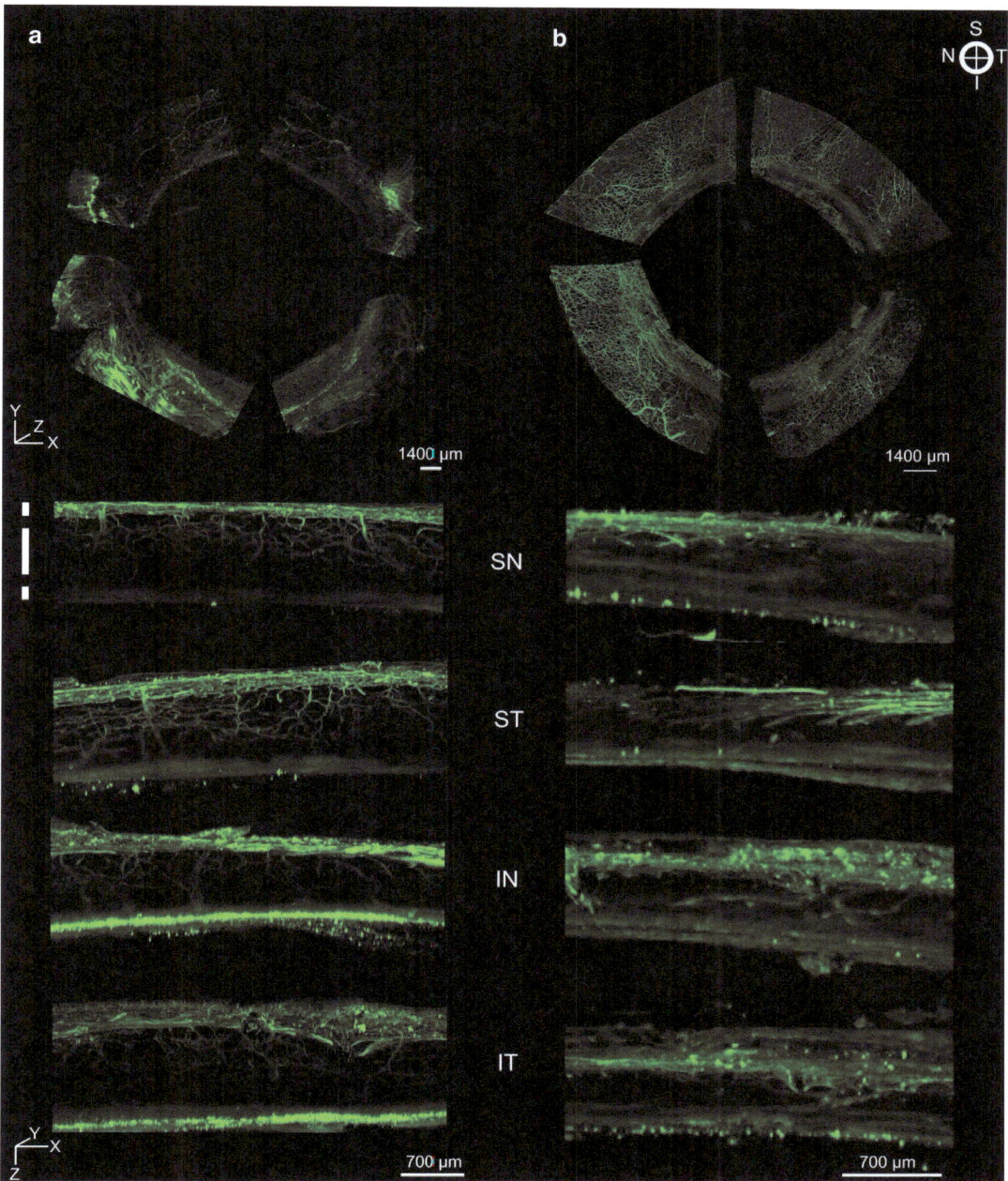

Fig. 7.7 Ribbon-scanning confocal microscopy reconstruction of the complete porcine (**a**, left) [69] and human (**b**, right) outflow tract. Bottom panels show angle view of each quadrant with distinct collector channel region (parallel to middle white line) communicating between the TM (bottom white line) and scleral vascular plexus (top white line)

several hours (Fig. 7.7a). Recently, outflow tracts of multiple human eyes have been similarly cleared, imaged, and reconstructed, revealing a variety of collector channel morphologies (Fig. 7.7b).

Time-resolved SD-OCT reconstructions demonstrated the ability of outflow tracts in ex vivo porcine eyes to dilate in response to the hypotensive nitric oxide and constrict responding to the hypertensive endothelin-1. Imaging data were supplemented with functional studies in which the TM was circumferentially removed and IOP responses of constant-rate perfusion cultures to nitric oxide were evaluated, correlating outflow tract vasodilation and increased outflow facility [70] (Fig. 7.8). University of Göttingen researcher

Hanna M. Gottschalk et al. used lipid emulsions as a contrast agent in OCT angiography (OCTA) of ex vivo porcine eyes, allowing time-resolved aqueous angiography [71]. The safety and efficacy of lipid emulsion use in patients have not yet been evaluated, although promising in conjunction with intraoperative OCT.

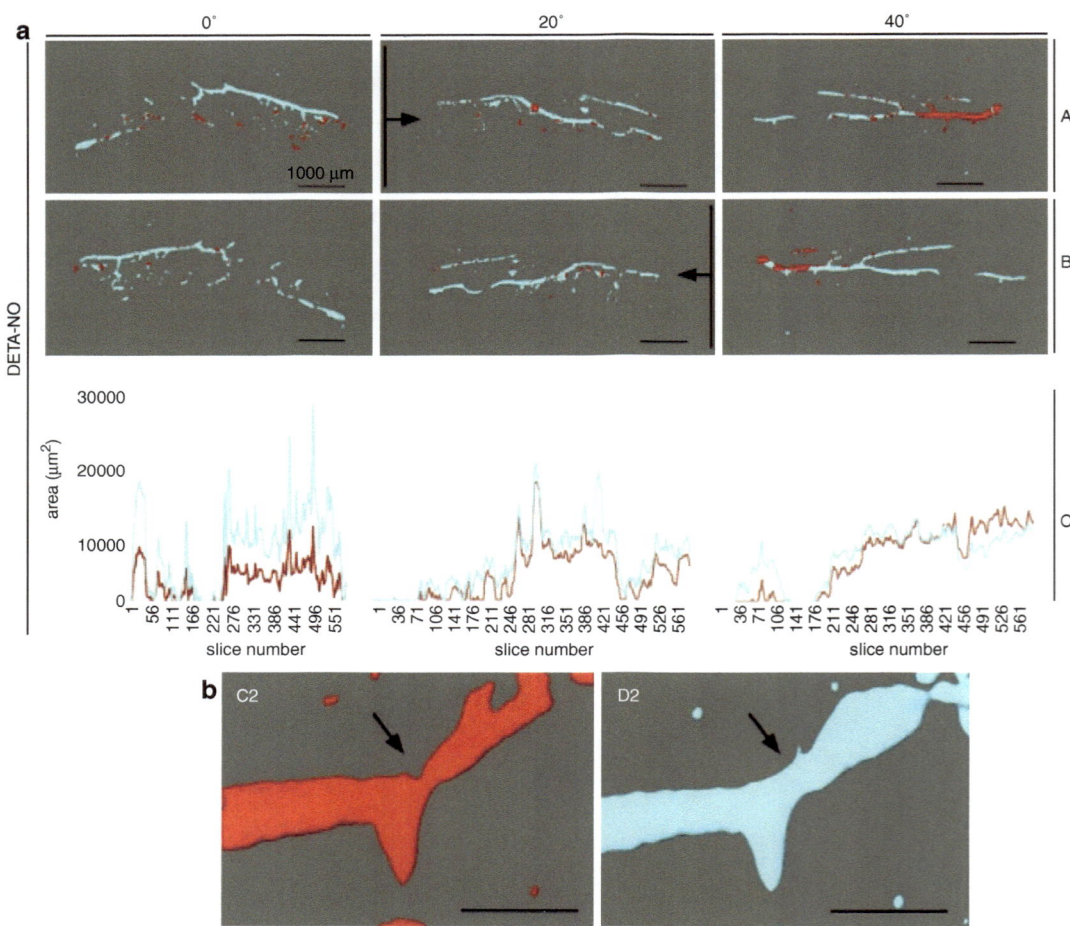

Fig. 7.8 (**a**) Quantification and of cross-sectional area pre- and posttreatment. Aligned and merged surface reconstructions taken with pretreatment pseudo-colored in red and posttreatment in cyan as viewed anteriorly ((A), A) and posteriorly ((A), B). DETA-NO-treated vessels show greater coverage with cyan, indicating a larger posttreatment than pretreatment intraluminal space (dilation).

CSA of virtual sections, made along the plane indicated by the black lines and in the direction of the black arrows, was calculated in silico. CSA was plotted throughout the length each sample ((A), C). (**b**) NO-induced focal dilation of outflow tract vessels. Outflow tract vessels pre- (C2, red) and posttreatment (D2, cyan) with DETA-NO vasodilator [70]

Outflow Computation and Simulation Using Depth Resolved Scan Data

Merely observing the perilimbal anatomy in glaucomatous eyes is not sufficient to understand the cause and location of post-trabecular outflow resistance. To show causality, it is necessary to demonstrate that a narrowed, closed, or otherwise altered vessel is capable of impacting the intraocular pressure. In theory, the change of a vessel's diameter has a powerful impact on outflow resistance that follows a fourth power rather than squared relation. For example, in theory, 6% vasodilation could cause a 20% reduction in IOP, while 9% dilation causes a 30% reduction in IOP, etc. However, there are paramount challenges: aqueous is a non-Newtonian fluid with a variable content of particles of mostly red blood cells. Flow is influenced by the viscosity of the vessel content and, due to the additional content of blood cells, potentially impacted by the hematocrit and the viscoelastic properties of individual red blood cells as is the case in other capillary networks. The geometry of microvessels also affects blood flow behavior in microcirculation [72]. However, an absent or patent outflow channel lumen are two extreme endpoints of a spectrum.

A 3D volume subset of the ribbon scanning confocal image data set was used to generate a mesh for the computational fluid dynamics (CFD) analysis. Figure 7.9 shows the smoothed surface mesh of this subsection. In the computational fluid simulation (Abaqus/CFD 2016, SIMULIA, Providence, RI), the aqueous flow was assumed as steady, incompressible, and Newtonian fluid [73] with a pressure of 15 mmHg at the inlet (top of Fig. 7.9a) and 8 mmHg at the outlet (bottom of Fig. 7.9a).

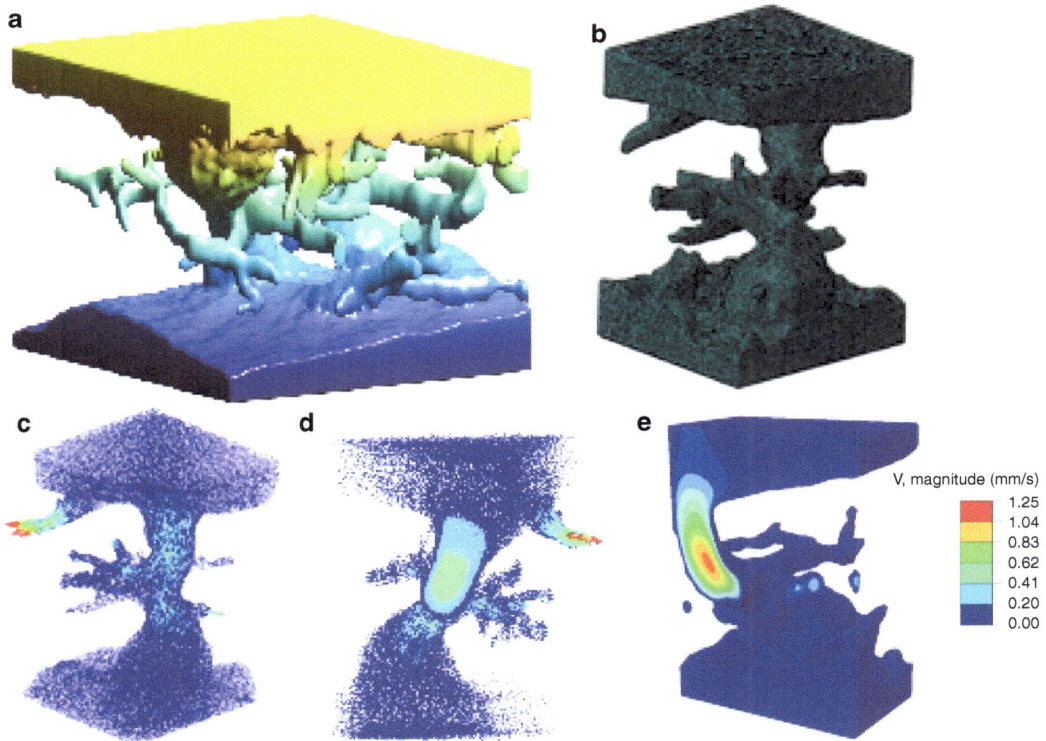

Fig. 7.9 Computational fluid dynamics (CFD) simulation of the flow within a small subsection of the anterior outflow pathway of a porcine eye acquired by ribbon scanning confocal microscopy. (**a**) Surface mesh after smoothing the geometry. (**b**) Final mesh for CFD simulation. (**c–e**) Velocity results from the CFD analysis

The computed velocity was 0.65 ± 0.32 mm/s with a range of 0–1.25 mm/s (panels c, d, and e of Fig. 7.9), which matches the flow speed in canalograms [7, 74].

Quantitative Outflow Imaging

Although outflow of aqueous humor can be estimated with fluorophotometry [75] and tonography [76], no method existed until recently to quantify segmental outflow at a given specific location in the outflow system. Cohan debated the lack of such outflow quantification already in 1958 and hoped to refine his radiopaque canalogram technique for this purpose [48]. The lack of an automated, standardized method to quantify aqueous humor outflow at a specific anatomic location

remained an obstacle to studying downstream outflow resistance elements [60] implicated in late failure of canal-based microincisional glaucoma surgeries [77]. It would also facilitate study of the outflow-enhancing effects of early cell [78] and gene therapy [79, 80] treatment strategies.

In 2014, current Johns Hopkins ophthalmology resident Bo Wang, MD, et al. used the Doppler effect of gold nanorods to estimate flow by optical coherence tomography [81] but later abandoned it because of poor spatial resolution and toxicity [82]. Qualitative fluorescein outflow studies in 1921 by E. Seidel [83] and G. Spital [84] led O. Benedikt in 1976 [85] to use the same dye to compute total outflow. He examined newly formed and preexisting vessels with appearance of lymphatic, venous, and primarily aqueous origin (Fig. 7.10). In

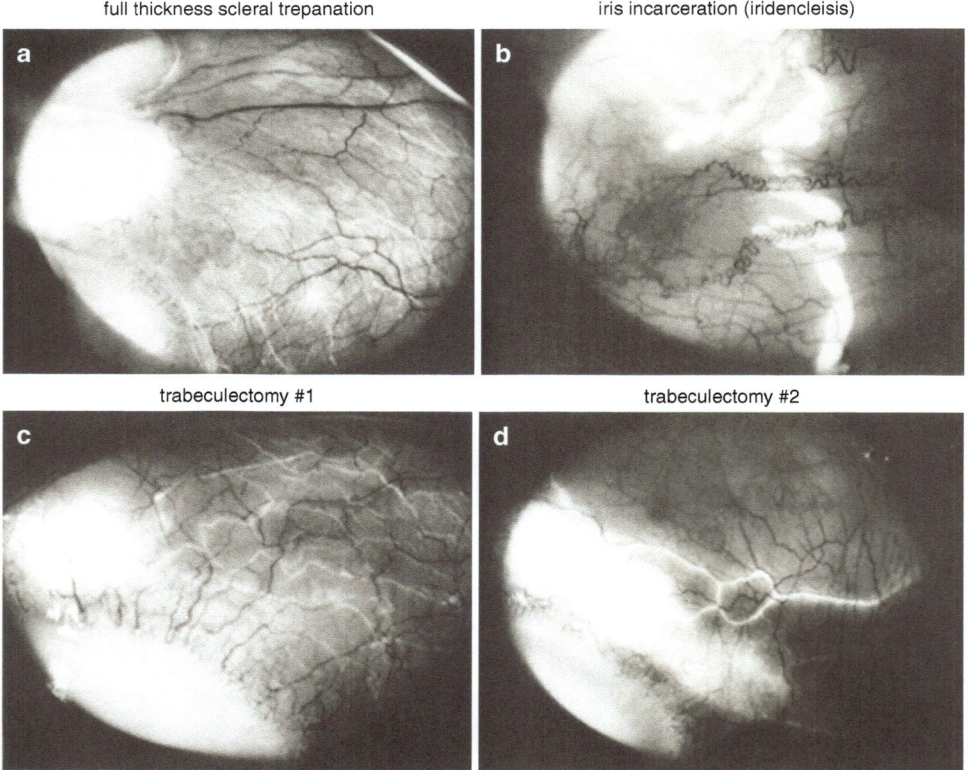

Fig. 7.10 Fluorescein outflow studies after full thickness trepanation (Elliot, (**a**)), full-thickness trepanation with iris incarceration (iridencleisis, (**b**)), and trabeculectomy ((**c**) and (**d**)). Percolation directly through the conjunctiva of the bleb (A), small lymphatic vessels ((**a**) and (**c**)), large lymphatic vessels with valves (**b**), and mostly aqueous venous (**d**) can be seen to drain aqueous. Seventeen out of 33 eyes had drainage vessels displaying lymphatic characteristics. (Courtesy of Dr. Benedikt) [85]

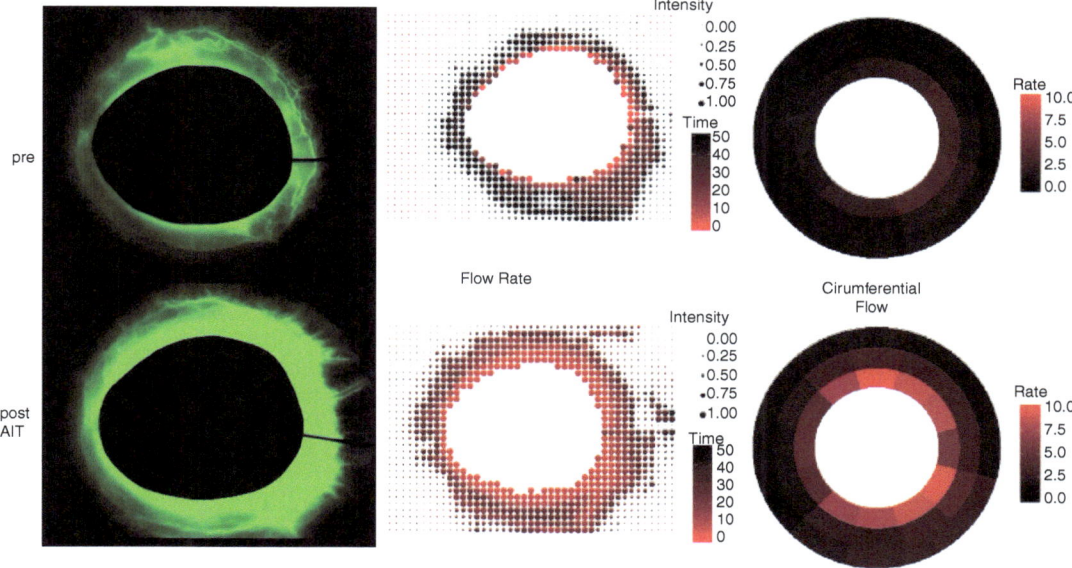

Fig. 7.11 Fluorescein canalograms (left, green) before (top) and after (bottom) outflow enhancement. Focal flow rates and intensity changes can be computed (middle) as well as perilimbal circumferential flow rates (right) [7]

2016, a "canalogram" method for regionally specific outflow measurement was developed (Fig. 7.11). Time-lapse fluorescence images were processed with open-source statistical software to evaluate circumferential as well as regional outflow [74]. Outflow patterns were found to change over time with the fastest flow nasally, which is the site of most surgical interventions. Perfusion of 0.5 μm fluorescent spheres allowed better definition of outflow structures for longer periods of time but necessitated removal of trabecular meshwork for proper microsphere passage [7]. These methods were adapted to reveal changes in outflow patterns following ab interno trabeculectomy in porcine eyes [6] and to evaluate trainee learning curves in a training model for glaucoma microsurgery [4]. Huang et al. utilized both fluorescein and indocyanine green (ICG) to detail dynamic flow in primate [86] and human eyes [87]. Similar to ex vivo porcine eyes, human angiographic signal was highest nasally.

Outlook

Technical options for outflow imaging exist on a spectrum of resolution and fidelity. With current methods, as resolution increases, the ability to measure function simultaneously is generally decreased. Fluorescein and ICG canalograms can measure regionally discrete outflow in real-time and can be conducted multiple times in each eye. However, leakage of tracer quickly limits definition of outflow tracts. Microbead canalograms greatly enhance the definition of vessels, allowing higher fidelity outflow quantification over time, but require bypass of the TM. Aggregating particulate load eventually alters physiology, rendering this a terminal experimental technique with currently available particles. Developing an agent that can pass the cornea noninvasively and at high enough of a concentration to be seen in the outflow system would facilitate clinical research into diagnostics that could be applied to identify patients suitable for microincisional glaucoma surgery focused on bypassing or removing the TM.

SD-OCT provides depth-resolved structural imaging without the need for non-physiologic contrast agents. Signal drop off in high-scattering scleral tissue often prevents full-thickness imaging with the desired definition. Additionally, SD-OCT alone cannot measure outflow function and must be supplemented with other imaging techniques. Anterior segment OCTA currently requires perfusion of lipid emulsions with an unknown effect on TM physiology. The highest-resolution imaging techniques, such as ribbon-scanning confocal microscopy and TEM, require fixation and optical clearing or sectioning of tissue so are unsuitable for same-sample time-series outflow function experiments.

Outflow imaging has slowly advanced over the last two centuries and remains crucial to understanding the outflow tract in health and disease in order to evolve new therapeutic strategies. Advancing these techniques and technologies will help ophthalmologists to better understand the disease process in glaucoma and the role of the distal outflow tract in current and future treatments.

Compliance with Ethical Requirements Ralitsa T. Loewen, Susannah Waxman, Hirut Kollech, Jonathan Vande Geest, and Nils A. Loewen declare that they have no conflict of interest. No human or animal studies were carried out by the authors for this chapter.

References

1. Nau CB, Malihi M, McLaren JW, Hodge DO, Sit AJ. Circadian variation of aqueous humor dynamics in older healthy adults. Invest Ophthalmol Vis Sci. 2013;54(12):7623–9.
2. Grant WM. Experimental aqueous perfusion in enucleated human eyes. Arch Ophthalmol. 1963;69:783–801.
3. Mäepea O, Bill A. Pressures in the juxtacanalicular tissue and Schlemm's canal in monkeys. Exp Eye Res. 1992;54(6):879–83.
4. Dang Y, Waxman S, Wang C, et al. Rapid learning curve assessment in an ex vivo training system for microincisional glaucoma surgery. Sci Rep. 2017;7(1):1605.
5. Wang C, Dang Y, Waxman S, Xia X, Weinreb RN, Loewen NA. Angle stability and outflow in dual blade ab interno trabeculectomy with active versus passive chamber management. PLoS One. 2017;12(5):e0177238.
6. Parikh HA, Loewen RT, Roy P, Schuman JS, Lathrop KL, Loewen NA. Differential canalograms detect outflow changes from trabecular micro-bypass stents and Ab Interno trabeculectomy. Sci Rep. 2016;6:34705.
7. Loewen RT, Brown EN, Scott G, Parikh H, Schuman JS, Loewen NA. Quantification of focal outflow enhancement using differential canalograms. Invest Ophthalmol Vis Sci. 2016;57(6):2831–8.
8. Dang Y, Wang C, Shah P, et al. Outflow enhancement by three different ab interno trabeculectomy procedures in a porcine anterior segment model. Graefes Arch Clin Exp Ophthalmol. 2018; https://doi.org/10.1007/s00417-018-3990-0.
9. Bussel II, Kaplowitz K, Schuman JS, Loewen NA, Trabectome Study Group. Outcomes of ab interno trabeculectomy with the trabectome by degree of angle opening. Br J Ophthalmol. 2015;99(7):914–9.
10. Loewen RT, Roy P, Parikh HA, Dang Y, Schuman JS, Loewen NA. Impact of a glaucoma severity index on results of trabectome surgery: larger pressure reduction in more severe glaucoma. PLoS One. 2016;11(3):e0151926.
11. Bussel II, Kaplowitz K, Schuman JS, Loewen NA, Trabectome Study Group. Outcomes of ab interno trabeculectomy with the trabectome after failed trabeculectomy. Br J Ophthalmol. 2014; https://doi.org/10.1136/bjophthalmol-2013-304717.
12. Parikh HA, Bussel II, Schuman JS, Brown EN, Loewen NA. Coarsened exact matching of phaco-trabectome to trabectome in Phakic patients: lack of additional pressure reduction from phacoemulsification. PLoS One. 2016;11(2):e0149384.
13. Pajic B, Pajic-Eggspuehler B, Haefliger I. New minimally invasive, deep sclerotomy ab interno surgical procedure for glaucoma, six years of follow-up. J Glaucoma. 2011;20(2):109–14.
14. Singh D, Bundela R, Agarwal A, Bist HK, Satsangi SK. Goniotomy ab interno "a glaucoma filtering surgery" using the Fugo plasma blade. Ann Ophthalmol. 2006;38(3):213–7.
15. Pajic B, Pajic-Eggspuehler B, Haefliger I, Hafezi F. Long-term results of a novel minimally invasive high-frequency deep Sclerotomy Ab Interno surgical procedure for glaucoma. Eur Ophthal Rev. 2012;6(1):3–6.
16. Schlemm F. Bulbus oculi. In: Rust JN, editor. Theoretisch-Praktisches Handbuch Der Chirurgie: Mit Einschluss Der Syphilitischen Und Augen-Krankheiten; in Alphabetischer Ordnung, vol. 3. Chir. 264. Berlin: Enslin; 1830. p. 332–8.
17. Teichmann-Stawiarski LK. Das Saugadersystem Vom Anatomischen Standpunkte, vol. 4 Anat. 190 c. Leipzig: Engelmann; 1861.
18. Schwalbe G. Untersuchungen über die Lymphbahnen des Auges und ihre Begrenzungen. Arch Mikrosk Anat. 1870;6(1):261–362.
19. Leber T. Studien über den Flüssigkeitswechsel im Auge. Albrecht von Graefes Archiv für Ophthalmologie. 1873;19(2):87–185.

20. Kizhatil K, Ryan M, Marchant JK, Henrich S, John SWM. Schlemm's canal is a unique vessel with a combination of blood vascular and lymphatic phenotypes that forms by a novel developmental process. PLoS Biol. 2014;12(7):e1001912.

21. Aspelund A, Tammela T, Antila S, et al. The Schlemm's canal is a VEGF-C/VEGFR-3-responsive lymphatic-like vessel. J Clin Invest. 2014;124(9):3975–86.

22. Park D-Y, Lee J, Park I, et al. Lymphatic regulator PROX1 determines Schlemm's canal integrity and identity. J Clin Invest. 2014;124(9):3960–74.

23. Rochon-Duvigneaud A. Recherches anatomique sur l'angle de la chambre antérieure et le canal de Schlemm. Arch Ophthalmol. 1892;12:732–44.

24. Leber T. Der Circulus venosus Schlemmii stehtnicht in offener Verbindung mit der vorderen Augenkammer. Graefe's Arhiv für Ophthalmologie. 1895;41(1):235–80.

25. Gutmann G. Ueber die Natur des Schlemm'schen Sinus und seine Beziehungen zur vorderen Augenkammer. Graefe's Arhiv für Ophthalmologie. 1895;41(1):28–55.

26. Bentzen CF, Leber T. Über die Filtration aus der vorderen Kammer bei normalen und glaukomatösen Augen. Graefes Arch Clin Exp Ophthalmol. 1895;41(3):208–57.

27. Leber T. In: Graefe A, Sämisch T, editors. Die Zirkulations- und Ernährungsverhältnisse des Auges, vol. 2. Leipzig: Wilhelm Engelmann; 1903. p. 63.

28. Seidel E. Weitere experimentelle Untersuchungen über die Quelle und den Verlauf der intraokularen Saftströmung IX. Mitteilung. Über den Abfluß des Kammerwassers aus der vorderen Augenkammer. Albrecht von Graefes Archiv für Ophthalmologie. 1921;104(3–4):357–402.

29. Seidel E. Weitere experimentelle Untersuchungen über die Quelle und den Verlauf der intraokularen Saftströmung XVII. Mitteilung. Ein weiterer experimenteller Beweis für das Bestehen einer hydrostatischen Druckdifferenz zwischen Vorderkammer und Schlemmschem Kanal bzw. episkleralen Venen im normalen Auge. Albrecht von Graefes Archiv für Ophthalmologie. 1922;108(3–4):420–3.

30. Stübel A. Über die Lymphgefäße des Auges. Graefes Arhiv für Ophthalmologie. 1922;110(1–2):109–33.

31. Dvorak-Theobald G. Schlemm's canal: its anastomoses and anatomic relations. Trans Am Ophthalmol Soc. 1934;32:574–95.

32. Graves B. Certain clinical features of the normal limbus. Br J Ophthalmol. 1934;18(6):305–41.

33. Friedenwald JS. Circulation of the aqueous: V. Mechanism of Schlemm's canal. Arch Ophthalmol. 1936;16(1):65–77.

34. Loewenstein A. Lipoid droplets in the Episclera as a regular change with age. Ophthalmologica. 1940;100(6):345–50.

35. Ascher KW. Aqueous Veins. Am J Ophthalmol. 1942;25(11):1301–15.

36. Ascher KW, Spurgeon WM. Compression tests on aqueous veins of glaucomatous eyes; application of hydrodynamic principles to the problem of intraocular-fluid elimination. Am J Ophthalmol. 1949;32 Pt. 2(6):239–51.

37. de Vries S. De zichtbare afvoer van het kamerwater, 1947.

38. Goldmann H. Ueber Abflussdruck und Glasstabphänomen; zur Pathogenese des einfachen Glaukoms. Ophthalmologica. 1948;116(4–5):195–8.

39. Ashton N. Anatomical study of Schlemm's canal and aqueous veins by means of neoprene casts. Part I. Aqueous veins. Br J Ophthalmol. 1951;35(5):291–303.

40. Loewenstein A. The anterior draining system in the human eye. Ophthalmologica. 1951;122(5):257–82.

41. Greaves DP, Perkins ES. Aqueous Veins in Rabbits. Br J Ophthalmol. 1951;35(2):119–23. https://doi.org/10.1136/bjo.35.2.119.

42. Dvorak-Theobald. Further studies on the canal of Schlemm. Am J Ophthalmol. 1955;39(4):65–89. https://doi.org/10.1016/0002-9394(55)90154-9.

43. Teng CC, Katzin HM, Chi HH. Primary degeneration in the vicinity of the chamber angle∗. Am J Ophthalmol. 1957;43(2):193–203. https://doi.org/10.1016/0002-9394(57)92910-0.

44. Teng CC, Paton RT, Katzin HM. Primary degeneration in the vicinity of the chamber angle∗: as an etiologic factor in wide-angle glaucoma. Am J Ophthalmol. 1955;40(5):619–31.

45. Cohan BE. Aqueous humor outflow: an experimental study using radiopaque materials. I. Paracentesis technique, response evoked, and demonstration of pathway of outflow. AMA Arch Ophthalmol. 1956;55(6):792–9.

46. Baltin MM. Roentgenographic study of the drainage of the aqueous from the anterior chamber. Vestn oftalmol. 1945;24:14–9.

47. Francois J, Neetens A, Collette JM. Microradiographic study of the inner wall of Schlemm's canal. Am J Ophthalmol. 1955;40(4):491–500.

48. Cohan BE. Radiography of aqueous humor outflow. AMA Arch Ophthalmol. 1958;60(1):110–5.

49. Rohen JW, Rentsch FJ. Über den Bau des Schlemmschen Kanals und seiner Abflußwege beim Menschen. Albrecht von Graefes Arch Klin Ophthalmol. 1968;176(4):309–29.

50. Morrison JC, Fraunfelder FW, Milne ST, Moore CG. Limbal microvasculature of the rat eye. Invest Ophthalmol Vis Sci. 1995;36(3):751–6.

51. Camp JJ, Hann CR, Johnson DH, Tarara JE, Robb RA. Three-dimensional reconstruction of aqueous channels in human trabecular meshwork using light microscopy and confocal microscopy. Scanning. 1997;19(4):258–63.

52. Johnson M, Johnson DH, Kamm RD, DeKater AW, Epstein DL. The filtration characteristics of the aqueous outflow system. Exp Eye Res. 1990;50(4):407–18.

53. Alvarado J, Murphy C, Polansky J, Juster R. Age-related changes in trabecular meshwork cellularity. Invest Ophthalmol Vis Sci. 1981;21(5):714–27.

54. Matsumoto Y, Johnson DH. Trabecular meshwork phagocytosis in glaucomatous eyes. Ophthalmologica. 1997;211:147–52.

55. Alvarado J, Murphy C, Juster R. Trabecular meshwork cellularity in primary open-angle glaucoma and nonglaucomatous normals. Ophthalmology. 1984;91(6):564–79.

56. Hann CR, Vercnocke AJ, Bentley MD, Jorgensen SM, Fautsch MP. Anatomic changes in Schlemm's canal and collector channels in normal and primary open-angle glaucoma eyes using low and high perfusion pressures distal outflow pathway at low and high pressure. Invest Ophthalmol Vis Sci. 2014;55(9):5834–41.

57. Acott TS, Kelley MJ. Extracellular matrix in the trabecular meshwork. Exp Eye Res. 2008;86(4):543–61.

58. Alvarado JA, Yun AJ, Murphy CG. Juxtacanalicular tissue in primary open angle glaucoma and in nonglaucomatous normals. Arch Ophthalmol. 1986;104(10):1517–28.

59. Rohen JW, Futa R, Lutjen-Drecoll E. The fine structure of the cribriform meshwork in normal and glaucomatous eyes as seen in tangential sections. Invest Ophthalmol Vis Sci. 1981;21:574–85.

60. Schuman JS, Chang W, Wang N, de Kater AW, Allingham RR. Excimer laser effects on outflow facility and outflow pathway morphology. Invest Ophthalmol Vis Sci. 1999;40(8):1676–80.

61. Rosenquist R, Epstein D, Melamed S, Johnson M, Grant WM. Outflow resistance of enucleated human eyes at two different perfusion pressures and different extents of trabeculotomy. Curr Eye Res. 1989;8(12):1233–40.

62. Kagemann L, Wollstein G, Ishikawa H, et al. Identification and assessment of Schlemm's canal by spectral-domain optical coherence tomography. Invest Ophthalmol Vis Sci. 2010;51(8):4054–9.

63. Kagemann L, Wollstein G, Ishikawa H, et al. 3D visualization of aqueous humor outflow structures in-situ in humans. Exp Eye Res. 2011;93(3):308–15.

64. Francis AW, Kagemann L, Wollstein G, et al. Morphometric analysis of aqueous humor outflow structures with spectral-domain optical coherence tomography. Invest Ophthalmol Vis Sci. 2012;53(9):5198–207.

65. Kagemann L, Nevins JE, Jan N-J, et al. Characterisation of Schlemm's canal cross-sectional area. Br J Ophthalmol. 2014;98 Suppl 2(Suppl 2):ii10–4.

66. Kagemann L, Wang B, Wollstein G, et al. IOP elevation reduces Schlemm's canal cross-sectional area. Invest Ophthalmol Vis Sci. 2014;55(3):1805–9.

67. Hann CR, Bentley MD, Vercnocke A, Ritman EL, Fautsch MP. Imaging the aqueous humor outflow pathway in human eyes by three-dimensional micro-computed tomography (3D micro-CT). Exp Eye Res. 2011;92(2):104–11.

68. Gonzalez JM Jr, Ko MK, Hong Y-K, Weigert R, Tan JCH. Deep tissue analysis of distal aqueous drainage structures and contractile features. Sci Rep. 2017;7(1):17071.

69. Waxman S, Loewen RT, Dang Y, Watkins SC, Watson AM, Loewen NA. High-resolution, three-dimensional reconstruction of the outflow tract demonstrates segmental differences in cleared eyes. Invest Ophthalmol Vis Sci. 2018;59(6):2371–80.

70. Waxman S, Wang C, Dang Y, Hong Y. Structure–function changes of the porcine distal outflow tract in response to nitric oxide. Invest Ophthalmol Vis Sci. 2018. https://iovs.arvojournals.org/article.aspx?articleid=2707233.

71. Gottschalk HM, Wecker T, Khattab MH, et al. Lipid emulsion–based OCT angiography for ex vivo imaging of the aqueous outflow tract. Invest Ophthalmol Vis Sci. 2019;60(1):397–406.

72. Pries AR, Secomb TW, Gaehtgens P. Biophysical aspects of blood flow in the microvasculature. Cardiovasc Res. 1996;32(4):654–67.

73. Wang W, Qian X, Song H, Zhang M, Liu Z. Fluid and structure coupling analysis of the interaction between aqueous humor and iris. Biomed Eng Online. 2016;15(Suppl 2):133.

74. Loewen RT, Brown EN, Roy P, Schuman JS, Sigal IA, Loewen NA. Regionally discrete aqueous humor outflow quantification using fluorescein canalograms. PLoS One. 2016;11(3):e0151754.

75. Brubaker RF. Measurement with fluorophotometry: I. plasma binding. II. Anterior segment, and III. Aqueous humor flow. Graefes Arch Clin Exp Ophthalmol. 1985;222(4–5):190–3.

76. Feghali JG, Azar DT, Kaufman PL. Comparative aqueous outflow facility measurements by pneumatonography and Schiotz tonography. Invest Ophthalmol Vis Sci. 1986;27:1776–80.

77. Kaplowitz K, Schuman JS, Loewen NA. Techniques and outcomes of minimally invasive trabecular ablation and bypass surgery. Br J Ophthalmol. 2014;98(5):579–85.

78. Du Y, Yun H, Yang E, Schuman JS. Stem cells from trabecular meshwork home to TM tissue in vivo. Invest Ophthalmol Vis Sci. 2013;54(2):1450–9.

79. Khare PD, Loewen N, Teo W, et al. Durable, safe, multi-gene lentiviral vector expression in feline trabecular meshwork. Mol Ther. 2008;16(1):97–106.

80. Barraza RA, McLaren JW, Poeschla EM. Prostaglandin pathway gene therapy for sustained reduction of intraocular pressure. Mol Ther. 2010;18(3):491–501.

81. Wang B, Kagemann L, Schuman JS, et al. Gold nanorods as a contrast agent for Doppler optical coherence tomography. PLoS One. 2014;9(3):e90690.

82. Gabriele Sandrian M, Wollstein G, Schuman JS, et al. Inflammatory response to intravitreal injection of gold nanorods. Br J Ophthalmol. 2012;96(12):1522–9.

83. Seidel E. Weitere experimentelle Untersuchungen über die Quelle und den Verlauf der intraokularen Saftströmung VI. Mitteilung. Die Filtrationsfähigkeit, eine wesentliche Eigenschaft der Scleralnarben nach erfolgreicher Elliotscher Trepanation. Albrecht von Graefes Archiv für Ophthalmologie. 1921;104(1–2):158–61.

84. Spital G. Über das druckherabsetzende Prinzip der Elliotschen Scleraltrepanation beim chronischen Glaukom. Albrecht von Graefes Archiv für Ophthalmologie. 1921;106(1):187–94.

85. Benedikt O. Demonstration of aqueous outflow patterns of normal and glaucomatous human eyes through the injection of fluorescein solution in the anterior chamber (author's transl). Albrecht Von Graefes Arch Klin Exp Ophthalmol. 1976;199(1):45–67.

86. Huang AS, Li M, Yang D, Wang H, Wang N, Weinreb RN. Aqueous angiography in living nonhuman primates shows segmental, pulsatile, and dynamic angiographic aqueous humor outflow. Ophthalmology. 2017;124(6):793–803.

87. Huang AS, Penteado RC, Saha SK, et al. Fluorescein aqueous angiography in live normal human eyes. J Glaucoma. 2018;27(11):957–64.

Future Novel Imaging Methods

8

Mahnaz Shahidi and Anthony E. Felder

Introduction

Glaucoma is an ocular disease causing irreversible visual function loss. It is estimated more than 60 million people worldwide have glaucoma and its incidence is anticipated to increase to 76 million by 2020 and more than 111 million by 2040 [1]. Glaucoma causes damage to the optic nerve head (ONH) and is accompanied by loss of retinal ganglion cells (RGCs) and reduction in the visual field (VF) [2]. Although increased intraocular pressure (IOP) is considered a major risk factor for the development of glaucoma, there is supportive evidence for a role of ocular microcirculation in glaucoma pathophysiology [3–6]. It is thought that increased IOP may cause deformation of the lamina cribrosa (LC) within the ONH, thus blocking axonal transport and altering blood flow, which can impair cellular metabolic function and eventually lead to cell death. Currently, it is not known whether blood flow alteration and dysregulation are the primary cause or consequence of VF loss due to glaucoma. Clinically, imaging technologies have played an important role in visualizing abnormalities in the ONH structure and retinal cell layers due to glaucoma. The advent of novel optical imaging technologies with higher depth resolution, tissue penetration, and image acquisition rate has allowed quantitative evaluation of retinal anatomy and hemodynamics at cellular and capillary levels. Furthermore, the availability of multimodal imaging techniques for assessment of retinal metabolic function offer a new approach for advancing knowledge of glaucoma pathophysiology. Finally, application of image-based machine learning methods enables and improves screening, early detection, and progression monitoring of glaucomatous damage. In this chapter, imaging techniques and their application for quantitative assessment of retinal and ONH anatomy, blood flow, vascular oxygen content, oxygen metabolic rate, and use with artificial intelligence approaches are described.

Optical Coherence Tomography

Optical coherence tomography (OCT) is an imaging technique based on interferometry, where a broadband infrared light source is split into two arms: a reference and a sample. The interference between the reference beam and backscattered light from the retina generates an image of anatomical structures across the retinal depth. Application of OCT has revolu-

M. Shahidi (✉)
USC Roski Eye Institute, Keck Medicine of University of Southern California,
Los Angeles, CA, USA
e-mail: mshahidi@usc.edu

A. E. Felder
Richard & Loan Hill Department of Bioengineering,
University of Illinois at Chicago, Chicago, IL, USA

© Springer Nature Switzerland AG 2020
R. Varma et al. (eds.), *Advances in Ocular Imaging in Glaucoma*, Essentials in Ophthalmology,
https://doi.org/10.1007/978-3-030-43847-0_8

tionized clinical retinal imaging and allowed imaging and thickness measurement of cell layers, approaching in vivo optical biopsy of tissue [7–10]. In 1991, time-domain OCT imaging was first demonstrated, and in 1993, OCT images of the human optic disc and macula were generated [11–13]. Shortly thereafter, spectral domain OCT (SD-OCT) was introduced, which is based on the same principle as time-domain OCT, but the interferometry is performed in the Fourier-domain with the use of a high-speed spectrometer. With greater imaging speed and depth resolution offered by SD-OCT, real-time visualization and more accurate quantitative thickness measurement of individual retinal layers has been realized [14].

Imaging of Retinal Layer Thickness

SD-OCT imaging is extensively used for quantitative assessment of circumpapillary retinal nerve fiber layer (RNFL) and macular ganglion cell layer complex (GCC) thickness at stages of glaucoma [15, 16]. Moreover, recent studies evaluated the diagnostic power of retinal layer thickness for detection of glaucoma [17–21]. Specifically, the Advanced Imaging of Glaucoma Study showed diagnosis of glaucoma is improved by combining measurements of peripapillary RNFL and GCC thickness [22]. Furthermore, research shows changes in peripapillary RNFL and GCC depend on the stage of glaucoma. In fact, the most diagnosed parameters in early and severe glaucoma were shown to be RNFL and GCC thickness, respectively [23, 24]. Assessment of progressive longitudinal changes in retinal layer thickness offers another approach for glaucoma diagnosis as compared to classification of eyes based on normative databases [25]. Indeed, the Advanced Imaging for Glaucoma Study showed reductions in peripapillary RNFL and GCC thickness can predict the development of glaucomatous visual field (VF) loss in glaucoma suspects and pre-perimetric glaucoma patients [26]. Furthermore, changes in RNFL and GCC thickness were detected over time in normal tension glaucoma (NTG) [27]. Also, a temporal relationship between peripapillary RNFL and macular GCC thickness was reported, showing changes in the RGC layer thickness is detectable prior to a corresponding RNFL thickness change in early glaucoma [28].

Imaging of the Optic Nerve Head

Visualization of changes in the ONH is considered a hallmark in the clinical diagnosis of glaucoma. SD-OCT imaging has been used for assessment of ONH parameters based on visualization and quantitative measurement of the Bruch's membrane opening (BMO). Some studies have demonstrated improved evaluation of the optic disc margin and size by visualization of BMO [29, 30]. Recent assessment of neuroretinal rim tissue based on the BMO minimum rim width and area was reported. Figure 8.1 shows an example OCT B-scan through the ONH and the methodology for measurement of neuroretinal rim tissue by delineating BMO and inner limiting membrane [31]. By imaging the BMO, assessment of the neuroretinal rim and identification of biomarkers for early detection of glaucoma has been enhanced [29, 32–34]. Moreover, measurements of neuroretinal rim parameters derived from SD-OCT images were shown to be reproducible and better correlated with both RNFL thickness and VF loss than rim measurements within the BMO plane or the clinical disc margin [31, 35]. Other studies indicated adjustments for age and axial length are needed to ensure optimal glaucoma diagnosis based on BMO-based parameters [36–38]. The lamina cribrosa (LC) is a multilayered structure at the posterior of the ONH and thought to be the site of axonal injury in glaucoma. With recent advances in OCT imaging, it is possible to visualize the LC in human eyes. Specifically, SD-OCT images of the ONH have demonstrated LC deformation in glaucoma and LC tilt was shown to correlate with myopia and glaucoma [39, 40]. Furthermore, 3D maps of LC strain in response to acute elevation of IOP have indicated LC deformations may serve as biomarkers for predicting glaucomatous ONH damage [41].

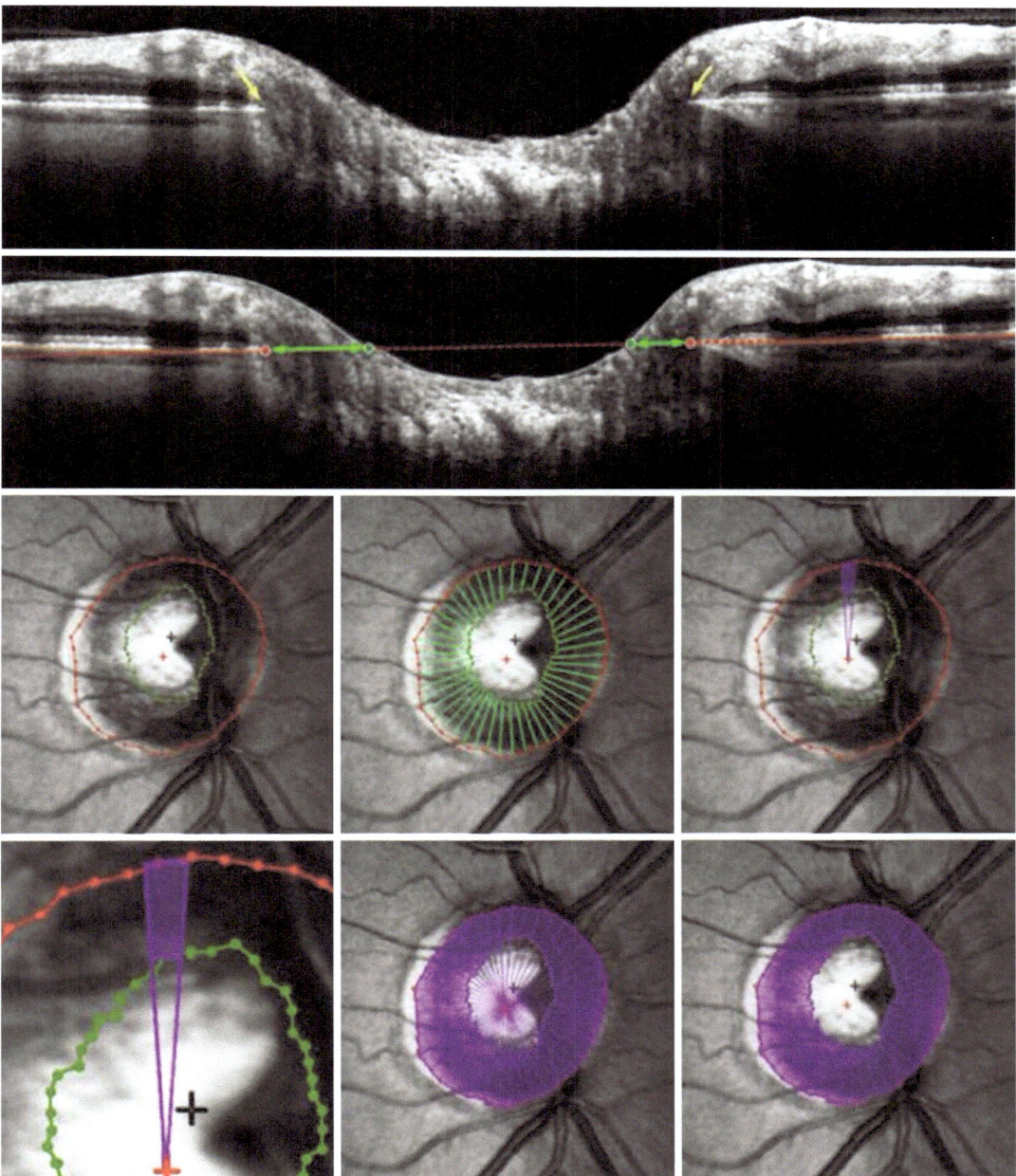

Fig. 8.1 An OCT B-scan image through the ONH and the methodology for measurement of neuroretinal rim tissue by delineating BMO and inner limiting membrane (ILM). Yellow arrows and red circles indicate the BMO and were used to define a red line on the B-scan, along which the intersections with ILM are shown in green circles. The BMO horizontal rim area (purple) was calculated as surface area between BMO and ILM. (Reprinted with permission from Gardiner et al., Ref. [31])

Enhanced Depth Imaging

In OCT imaging systems, the scattering of near-infrared light from the photoreceptors reduces the signal from deeper structures, namely, the choroid. In 2008, a new technique called enhanced depth imaging (EDI) was introduced to overcome this limitation and provide images of the choroid using a conventional SD-OCT system [42]. EDI has become a mode of SD-OCT

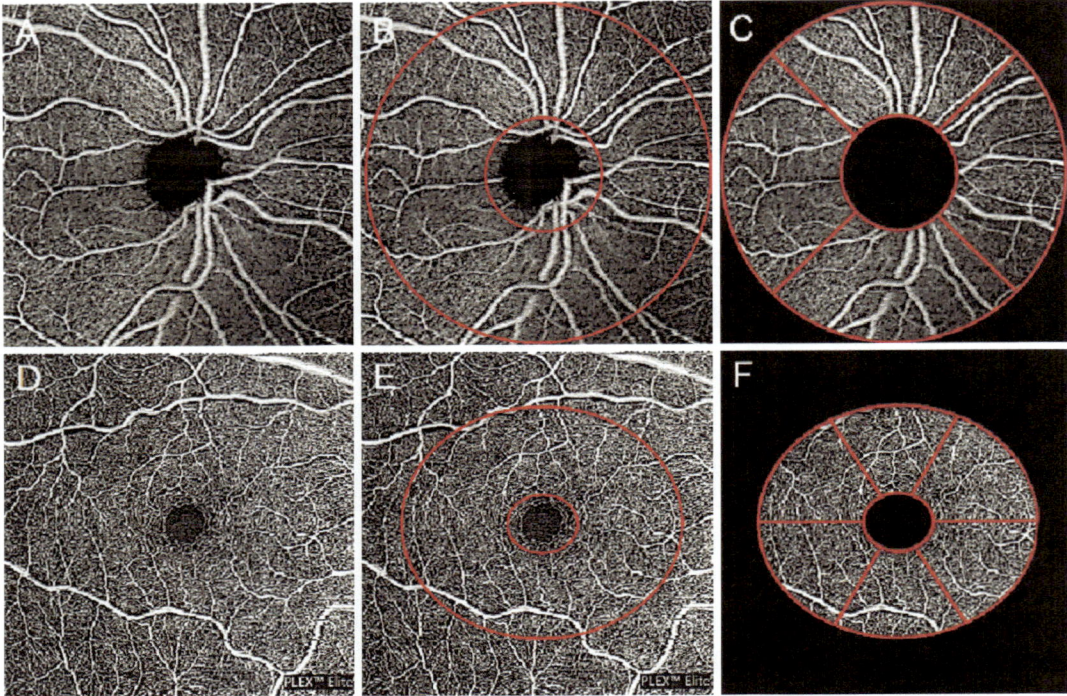

Fig. 8.2 OCTA images displaying retinal microvasculature in the ONH (**A–C**) and macula regions (**D–F**) with various regions of interest used for post-processing (red)

allowing improved visualization of the deeper structures of the retina and ONH based on an inverted image with the light source focused on the choroid. The use of EDI has determined a reduction in choroidal thickness due to glaucoma and changes with respect to intraocular pressure (IOP) and visual sensitivity [43–46]. In addition, EDI has been applied to demonstrate associations between cup depth, LC, and prelaminar neural tissue thickness [47]. In fact, a longitudinal study using EDI showed a deeper and thinner LC, and focal LC defects were related to the rate of RNFL thinning [48].

Imaging of the Vasculature

OCT angiography (OCTA) is a noninvasive imaging technique for assessment of capillary perfusion and microvascular density in the peripapillary and macular regions. It detects variations in the intensity or phase of the optical signal due to the motion of red blood cells within

the vasculature from repeated scans acquired at high rates in the same retinal location. Figure 8.2 shows OCTA images of the retinal microvasculature in the macula and ONH [49]. The clinical application of OCTA for detection of perfusion abnormalities due to glaucoma has been described [15, 50–55]. Specifically, OCTA has been applied to visualize changes in peripapillary and macular perfusion in glaucoma, as well as age-related changes in vessel density [49, 56, 57]. Furthermore, an association between peripapillary and macular vessel density has been established in glaucoma suspects and subjects [58]. Other studies have reported alterations in the density of peripapillary capillaries in glaucoma suspects and at stages of glaucoma [59–67]. Moreover, longitudinal studies demonstrated the rate of change in the capillary density over time was higher in glaucoma as compared to glaucoma suspects [68]. The relationship between vessel density and VF loss due to glaucoma has been reported, and reduced peripapillary vessel density was shown to correspond with VF loss and LC defects [69–72]. Interestingly, peripapillary and macular vascular densities were shown to be decreased in the unaffected hemifields of glaucomatous eyes with one affected hemifield [73].

Imaging of Blood Flow

Since impairments of ocular blood flow and its regulation have been proposed to have a role in glaucoma [74], imaging methods have been developed and applied for assessment of blood flow in glaucoma [51, 75, 76]. Laser Doppler flowmetry is a method that measures the Doppler shift of light scattered by the moving red blood cells based on the Fourier analysis of beating frequencies [77]. Using this method, abnormal autoregulation of ONH blood flow was reported in primary open angle glaucoma (POAG) [78]. Moreover, retinal capillary blood flow was shown to be increased with antioxidant supplementation, further supporting a role of microcirculation in glaucoma [79]. In contrast, retrobulbar blood velocity measured by color Doppler imaging was shown to be useful for discriminating pre-perimetric from healthy subjects and for monitoring glaucoma progression [80–83]. Additionally, blood velocity was shown to correlate with structural changes in the ONH and macular thickness over time in OAG. A longitudinal study demonstrated an association of ophthalmic artery blood flow velocity with structural and functional glaucoma progression [84].

The Doppler technique has also been incorporated into OCT imaging systems to measure retinal blood flow using various approaches [85–90]. To minimize the error associated with angle determination in Doppler OCT systems, dual-angle Doppler OCT and dual-beam OCT systems were developed [90–95]. Application of Doppler OCT has shown reduced retinal blood flow was associated with thinner RNFL and GCC [96]. This study also reported retinal blood flow was reduced in hemifields with VF loss, as well as in the perimetrically normal hemisphere of glaucomatous eyes. Recently, an en face Doppler approach for high-speed OCT systems

that eliminated the need for angle calculation was introduced to measure the high axial blood velocity in the central retinal vasculature [97–99]. This method was also applied to measure blood flow in retinal vessel branches with lower speed conventional OCT systems by employing tilted or multiple en face planes [100, 101]. Studies have shown retinal blood flow measured by Doppler OCT is reduced in glaucoma subjects [101, 102].

Laser speckle flowgraphy (LSFG) is a method to measure relative blood flow based on interference or speckle patterns generated from the scattering of coherent light by the movement of blood. LSFG was first demonstrated in 1981 and later developed for assessment of ONH blood flow [103, 104]. With this technique, blood flow is reported in arbitrary units of blur, and software algorithms were developed to analyze the mean blur pulse waveform and derive other indices [105, 106]. Mean blur rate (MBR) measured by LSFG was shown to be related to mitochondria dysfunction in subjects with severe OAG and associated with impaired vasoreactive response to hyperoxia in POAG [107, 108]. Furthermore, abnormalities in ONH blood flow are thought to be involved in the pathogenesis of NTG [3]. The findings of a close relationship between MBR, RNFL thickness, visual sensitivity, and systemic markers of oxidative stress suggest that oxidative stress is associated with decreased blood flow in NTG [109]. Moreover, a correlation between MBR and GCC thickness was reported in eyes with untreated NTG and hemifield defect, suggesting that a reduction in ONH microcirculation may be an early indicator for the presence and progression of glaucoma [110]. In addition, MBR and LSFG measurements of waveform changes in ONH blood flow were shown to differentiate NTG and healthy subjects and identify early glaucoma [111–113]. MBR was also shown to be a significant contributor to a right-left difference in VF defect in NTG and predictive of VF loss progression [114, 115]. Furthermore, MBR was shown to be an independent factor affecting reduction in circumpapillary RNFL thickness and VF in pre-perimetric glaucoma [116].

Optical Coherence Tomography with Swept Laser Source

Swept source OCT (SS-OCT) is a Fourier-domain imaging modality, similar to SD-OCT, but instead uses a tunable laser light source with a longer central wavelength compared to SD-OCT. Consequently, SS-OCT allows imaging of deeper retinal and ONH structures. Figure 8.3 shows examples of B-scans through the ONH generated with both SD-OCT and SS-OCT [117]. The higher image acquisition rate and wider-field scanning advantages of SS-OCT for detection of pre-perimetric and early perimetric glaucoma, visualization of ONH structures, and evaluation of the RNFL defects have been demonstrated [117–120]. In addition, SS-OCT images of the ONH have been analyzed for measurement of BMO and LC structural parameters and for quantitative 3D evaluation of the LC microstructures [81, 121–123]. SS-OCT imaging has also been applied for improved visualization of the anterior eye structures and macular capillary network [124–127].

Optical Coherence Tomography with Visible Laser

An emerging technology is visible light OCT (vis-OCT), which is also based on low coher-ence interferometry in the Fourier-domain, but uses a broadband light source spanning the visible spectrum [128–130]. In addition to providing volumetric, high-resolution imaging of the retina, vis-OCT also permits quantitative determination of hemoglobin concentrations [131, 132]. The vis-OCT technology shows promise for assessment of elastic light scattering properties of retinal cell layers, specifically the RNFL [133]. In addition, vis-OCT is capable of measuring retinal vessel hemoglobin oxygen saturation by oximetry [134–136]. An important feature is that vis-OCT systems allow combined hemoglobin oxygen saturation and blood flow measurements to determine the rate of oxygen metabolism [137, 138]. With this new technology, cell elasticity and oxygen metabolism measures can complement conventional anatomical features with promise to improve prediction of glaucoma development.

Adaptive Optics Imaging

Retinal image quality is degraded by the presence of both low-order (e.g., defocus and astigmatism) and high-order (e.g., spherical and coma) ocular aberrations, limiting the ability to resolve retinal features at a cellular level. Adaptive optics (AO) is a technique that compensates for these aberrations and may be integrated into existing retinal imaging modalities, thereby improving lateral

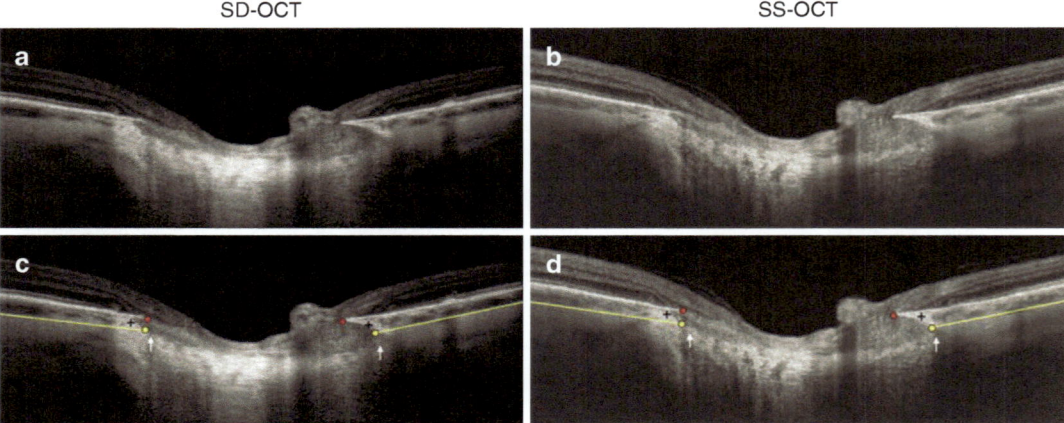

Fig. 8.3 OCT B-scan images through the ONH generated with both SD-OCT (**a** and **c**) and SS-OCT (**b** and **d**). The BMO (red dot), posterior choroid (yellow line), bor-der tissue from the sclera to Bruch's membrane (black crosshair), LC insertions (white arrow), and anterior sclera canal opening (yellow dot) are indicated

and axial resolution of retinal images. The general scheme for integrating AO into retinal imaging systems involves the accommodation of two additional optical components: (1) a wavefront sensor and (2) a deformable mirror to compensate for the detected wavefront aberrations. AO is primarily incorporated in three retinal imaging systems: the scanning laser ophthalmoscope (SLO), the flood illumination ophthalmoscope (FIO), and OCT. Figure 8.4 illustrates improvement in resolution with the use of AO incorporated in SLO, FIO, and OCT imaging systems.

Adaptive Optics in the Scanning Laser Ophthalmoscope

Clinically, fundus examination and photography were sufficient to qualitatively evaluate ONH changes, cupping, and RNFL defects in glaucoma, but quantitative evaluation was precluded [139, 140]. In the late 1980s, the confocal SLO was introduced and used to image retinal tissue in human eyes [141–143]. Compared to fundus examination, SLO demonstrated better depth discrimination and could quantitatively evaluate certain retinal anatomical structures [144–146]. However, the SLO's depth resolution was limited, precluding quantified measurement of individual retinal cell layers [147].

In 1989, AO was first used in combination with a SLO (AOSLO) to improve both axial and lateral resolution of retinal images [148]. This implementation used an active 13-electrode deformable mirror array, relay lenses, and linear stage to correct low-order wavefront aberrations as measured by conventional refractometry. In 1994, a Shack-Hartmann wavefront sensor was used to objectively measure ocular aberrations in human eyes [149]. The Shack-Hartmann sensor is comprised of an array of lenses—lenslets—mated with a camera to detect high-order wavefront aberrations. When paired with a deformable mirror, it can be used for wavefront aberration correction. Since then, advancements in AOSLO have further improved resolution and enabled real-time visualization of the retinal tissue at a cellular level [150–159].

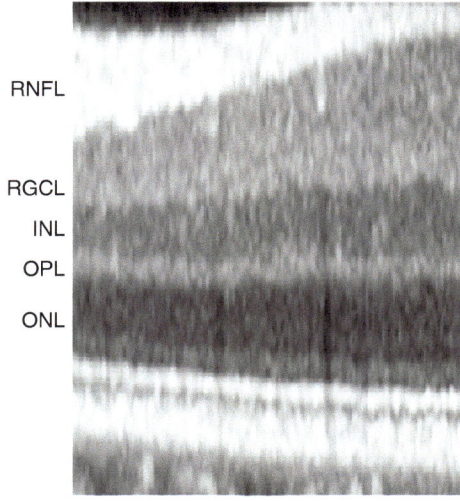

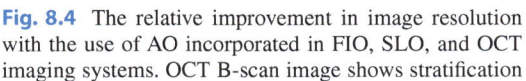

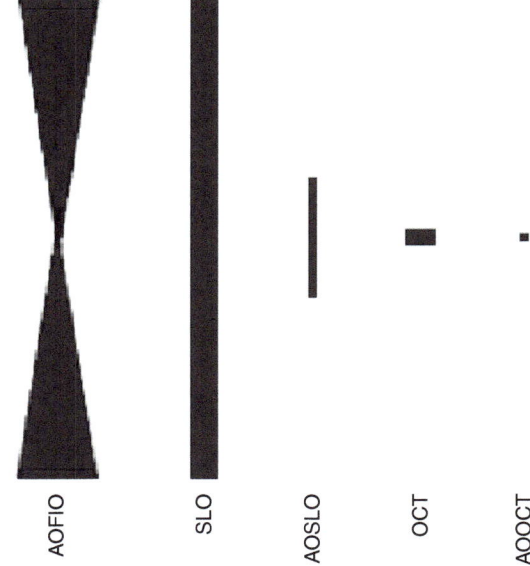

Fig. 8.4 The relative improvement in image resolution with the use of AO incorporated in FIO, SLO, and OCT imaging systems. OCT B-scan image shows stratification and thickness of individual retinal cell layers relative to imaging resolutions

AOSLO has been used to discern glaucomatous damage in RNFL fibers since it was difficult to image by OCT [160]. Other studies using AOSLO examined the RNFL near fixation and the temporal raphe, establishing these regions as early predictors for glaucomatous damage [161, 162]. AOSLO is also capable of reproducibly assessing the LC, revealing early glaucomatous damage in morphology and increased pore area in both human glaucoma and nonhuman primate models of glaucoma [163–166]. In addition to imaging the ONH, AOSLO is used to image individual cells of interest in glaucoma, such as RGCs [167]. Several studies have imaged photoreceptors and rhodopsin in human eyes [159, 168, 169], as well as assessed cone photoreceptor integrity in glaucoma [170]. Interestingly, one study reported swelling of the photoreceptors in glaucoma using AOSLO [171].

Adaptive Optics in the Flood Illumination Ophthalmoscope

In 1997, the first closed-loop AO system for a fundus camera was described [172]. This system incorporated a Shack-Hartmann sensor in combination with a 37-actuator deformable mirror to correct both low- and high-order wavefront aberrations and generated images of cone photoreceptor distribution. However, image acquisition rate was low, precluding real-time application. In 2001, real-time AO fundus camera systems were first introduced [150, 173]. With commercially available AO flood illumination ophthalmoscope (AOFIO), photoreceptor and microvascular changes due to disease have been investigated [174–176]. One glaucoma study demonstrated a blue-yellow defect in retinal cone photoreceptors using an AO fundus camera [177]. Other studies reported dark regions in the cone photoreceptor mosaic corresponding to areas of decreased visual sensitivity in glaucomatous eyes [178, 179]. AOFIO has also been used to image the lamina cribrosa and reveal changes to pore morphology [180].

Adaptive Optics in Optical Coherence Tomography

In 2005, AO was incorporated into OCT imaging systems (AOOCT), demonstrating superior spatial resolution compared to conventional OCT [181–185]. Today, AOOCT provides greater knowledge of changes in retinal cell morphology and ONH structure due to glaucoma. Figure 8.5 presents an AOOCT volume of retinal tissue with examined en face images of retinal cell layers [186]. Several studies have reported the use of AOOCT to image the RNFL, permitting visualization of individual fibers [160, 187, 188]. Also, AOOCT enabled the study of LC microstructure by generation of 3D reconstructions [189]. With the improved spatial resolution of AOOCT, imaging of the ONH and retina at the cellular level was recently demonstrated, particularly in RGCs, which have been difficult to image due to their inherent transparency [190–193].

Fluorescence Imaging

In fluorescence imaging, a single photon is absorbed by a fluorophore's electron to transition the molecule from its ground state to an excited state. This energy is released nearly instantly through the emission of a less energetic photon. In glaucoma research, fluorescence imaging has been used for evaluation of RGCs, including assessment of their neural activity and evaluation of their death. In vivo imaging of RGCs has been achieved by several fluorescence-based labeling techniques, including retrograde staining, transgenic models, and viral vectors [194]. Retrograde labeling is currently the most established of these techniques and has been used in conjunction with modified epifluorescence and scanning laser ophthalmoscope imaging systems to visualize RGCs in live rodents [195, 196]. In these studies, time-lapse and longitudinal assessment of RGCs was performed to circumvent both intra- and inter-animal variations and establish RGC quantification as a useful metric for evaluation of experimental

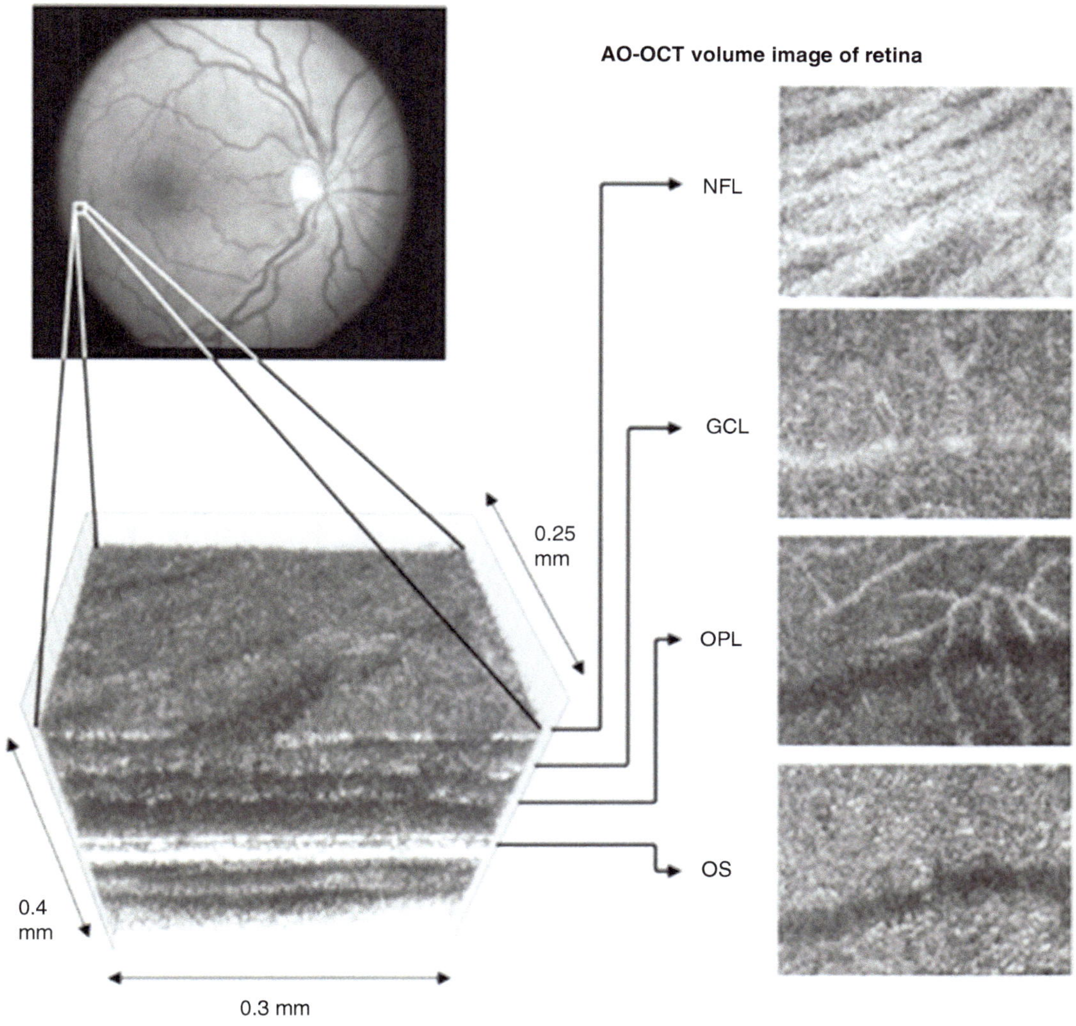

AO-OCT volume image of retina

NFL

GCL

OPL

OS

0.25 mm

0.4 mm

0.3 mm

Fig. 8.5 A retinal tissue image volume generated by AOOCT, displaying *en face* images of individual retinal cell layers. (Reprinted with permission from Miller et al., Ref. [186])

models of disease [197]. Figure 8.6 shows fluorescence images generated by retrograde labeling to monitor RGCs in vivo over time [195]. Other studies utilized calcium-indicator fluorescence dyes to assess the functional activity of RGCs [198–201]. Similarly, calcium imaging has been performed using transgenic techniques and viral vectors to study experimental animal models [199, 202, 203]. Neural activity has also been imaged using voltage-sensitive fluorescence dyes,

although this technique has not yet been demonstrated in the retina [204–206]. Another application of fluorescence imaging is real-time detection of apoptosing retinal cells (DARC), which has been specifically applied to assess RGC loss in glaucoma [207]. This technique relies on intravitreal injected fluorophore conjugated to annexin 5, which is a common protein for labelling apoptotic cells [208, 209]. DARC has recently been used in human eyes to demonstrate increased RGC apop-

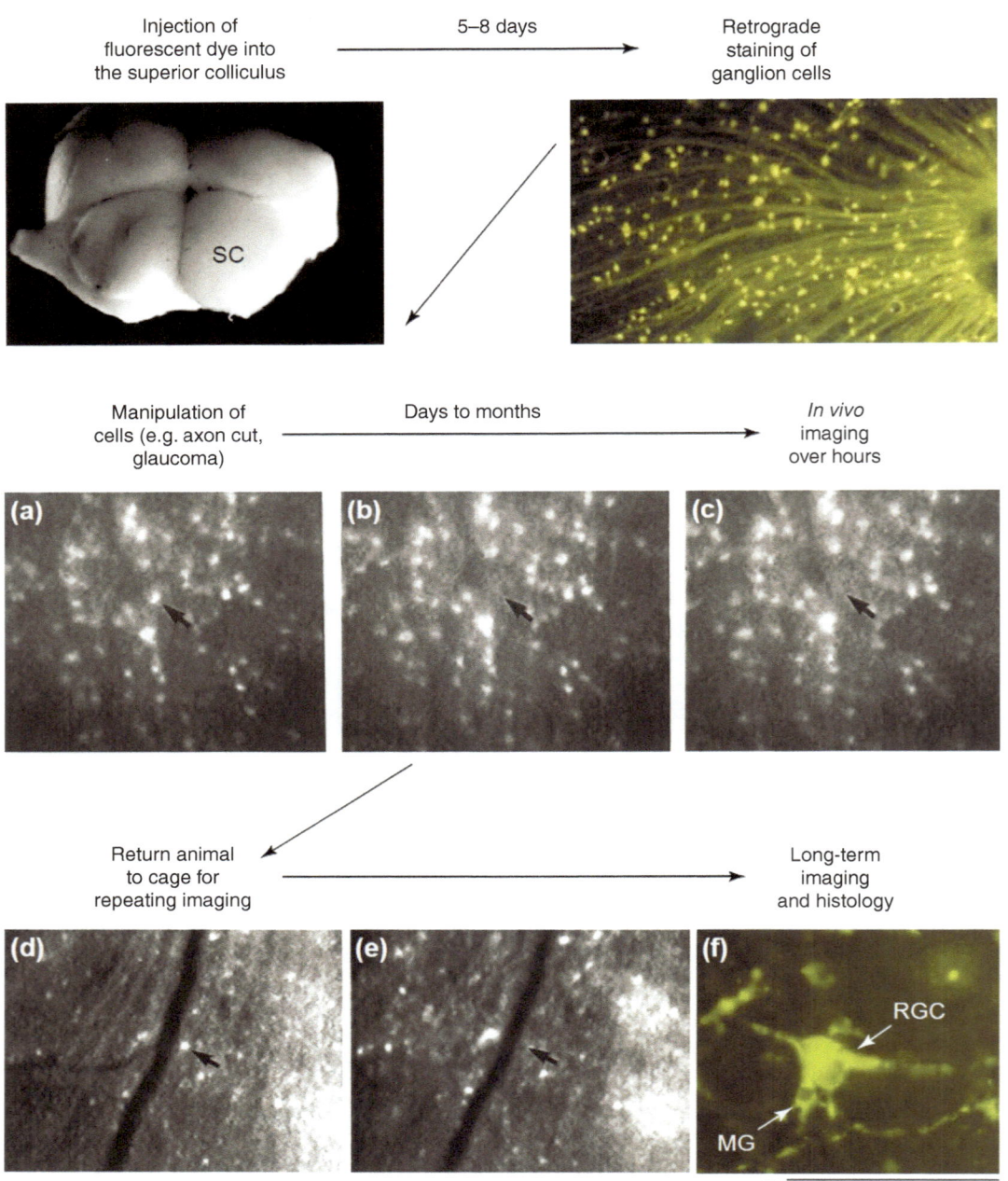

TRENDS in Neurosciences

Fig. 8.6 Time-lapse in vivo images of fluorescently labeled RGCs following retrograde staining. In vivo imaging of RGCs and their disappearance after injury (**a–e**), and maximal resolution of an RGC with attached microglial cell (**f**). (Reprinted with permission from Thanos et al., Ref. [195])

tosis in glaucoma subjects compared to healthy control subjects [210, 211].

There are also endogenous fluorophores within the ocular tissue that exhibit fluorescence in a process commonly referred to as autofluorescence. Retinal autofluorescence imaging primarily targets lipofuscin (A2E fluorophore) located in the retinal pigment epithelium (RPE). In addition to the detection of fluorescence intensity, the exponential decay of fluorescence over time may also be measured using a technique known as fluorescence lifetime imaging (FLIM) [212]. Fluorescence lifetime is a signature unique to each fluorophore and can be affected by localized chemical species, providing information on the microenvironment surrounding the fluorophore [213]. A notable application of FLIM is for the assessment of cellular energy metabolic state by measuring changes in fluorescence lifetimes of intracellular autofluorescent molecules like nicotinamide adenine dinucleotide (NADH) and flavin adenine dinucleotide (FAD). The use of FLIM for studying lipofuscin, FAD, and advanced glycation end products has been demonstrated in the human retina [214]. Furthermore, FLIM has also been used to demonstrate changes in macular fluorescence lifetime parameters due to glaucoma [215].

Two-Photon Fluorescence Imaging

Nonlinear processes in which two or more photons simultaneously interact with matter (i.e., multiphoton processes) may also be utilized for imaging. The simplest multiphoton processes involve the interactions of two photons, such as two-photon fluorescence (2PF) and second harmonic generation (SHG) imaging. 2PF is similar to conventional fluorescence, except two photons are simultaneously absorbed by a fluorophore's electron, whose relaxation emits a single photon of nearly twice the energy of the single excitation photon. SHG occurs in a non-centrosymmetric medium in which the two incident photons are annihilated by scattering to produce a third distinct photon at exactly twice the energy of the single excitation photon. Common to both 2PF and SHG techniques are photons of lower energy—or equivalently, light at a longer wavelength—are used to generate an optical signal with a higher energy or shorter wavelength of light. For example, near-infrared light is commonly used to elicit 2PF in the visible spectrum, with the benefit of providing deeper penetration into biological tissues and the ability to probe tissues in which transmission of short wavelength light is precluded. Since both 2PF and SHG are nonlinear optical processes, they require sufficiently high input light intensities and thus rely on excitation light commonly provided by a mode-locked, short-pulse laser source paired to a high numerical aperture lens. Notably, 2PF and SHG imaging intrinsically demonstrate high spatial and depth resolution since these nonlinear processes only occur within a portion of the focal imaging volume.

To date, 2PF imaging has only been demonstrated in animal models of glaucoma or explanted human tissues due to technical limitations and safety concerns. In animal models, 2PF and SHG have been used to assess the trabecular meshwork (TM) and the aqueous outflow system in enucleated eyes [216–218]. As shown in Fig. 8.7, 2PF imaging displayed heterogeneous global strain and changes in astrocyte orientation at the ONH within hours of sustained elevated IOP in mice [219]. Recently, 2PF was coupled with FLIM to demonstrate imaging of RPE in mice [220]. Evaluation of the anterior segment by 2PF and SHG imaging has also been performed in human corneal buttons [221]. Other studies imaged endogenous fluorescence mol-

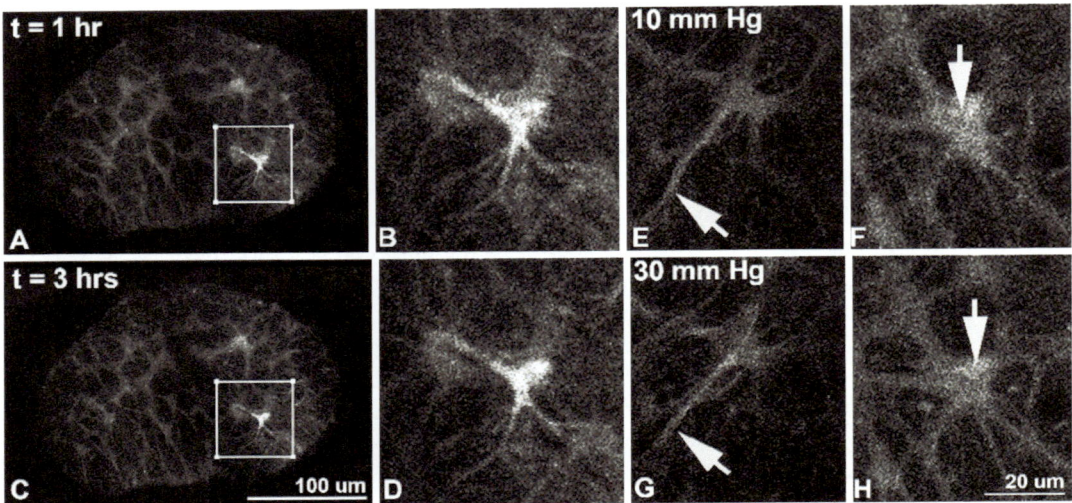

Fig. 8.7 Images of astrocytes at the ONH acquired by 2PF imaging (**A** and **C** under low magnification, **B** and **D** under high magnification) show changes in their shape and process orientation with elevated IOP (**E** and **F** at 10 mmHg, **G** and **H** at 30 mmHg)

ecules in corneoscleral rims to study the TM extracellular matrix and constituent components [222–224]. A related study utilized 2PF to identify several markers of glaucoma pathogenesis in the TM by imaging extracellular matrix interactions [225]. Imaging of human TM cell cultures allowed assessment of cellular metabolic activity through nicotinamide adenine dinucleotide phosphate [226]. Multiphoton techniques have also been used to demonstrate reduced RGC density in postmortem glaucomatous retinal samples [227].

Retinal Oximetry

Dual Wavelength Oximetry

Oximetry is a noninvasive optical imaging technique based on spectrophotometry that utilizes the difference in absorption spectra between oxygenated and deoxygenated hemoglobin to determine the oxygen saturation of hemoglobin (SO_2) in blood [228, 229]. Introduced in the late 1990s, dual wavelength retinal oximetry is commonly performed today, wherein reflectance images of the retina are acquired at two specific wavelengths of light [230]. From these images, an optical den-

sity ratio is calculated in retinal vessels and converted to SO_2 through empirical calibration [229, 231–233]. Notably, retinal images acquired for oximetry can also be analyzed to determine retinal vessel caliber and provide further information on vascular hemodynamics [234, 235].

The use of oximetry for the assessment of retinal arterial and venous SO_2 (SO_{2A} and SO_{2V}) has been of interest in glaucoma research [209]. Figure 8.8 shows examples of retinal vascular SO_2 maps generated in healthy (left) and glaucoma (right) subjects [236]. Current studies found increases in SO_{2V} and accompanying decreases in the arterial-venous SO_2 difference (SO_{2AV}) in glaucoma [236–239]. The increase in SO_{2V} correlated with VF loss, suggesting a relationship between glaucomatous damage, vision loss, and retinal oxygen extraction impairment [238]. Other studies commented on the relationship between glaucomatous structural damage and oximetry. Specifically, an inverse relationship between SO_{2V} and RNFL thickness was demonstrated [237], whereas no such correlation was confirmed in another study [240]. A reduction in retinal vessel caliber has been reported in glaucoma, sometimes in correlation with RNFL thickness, although some studies were not able to confirm this finding [239, 241–246].

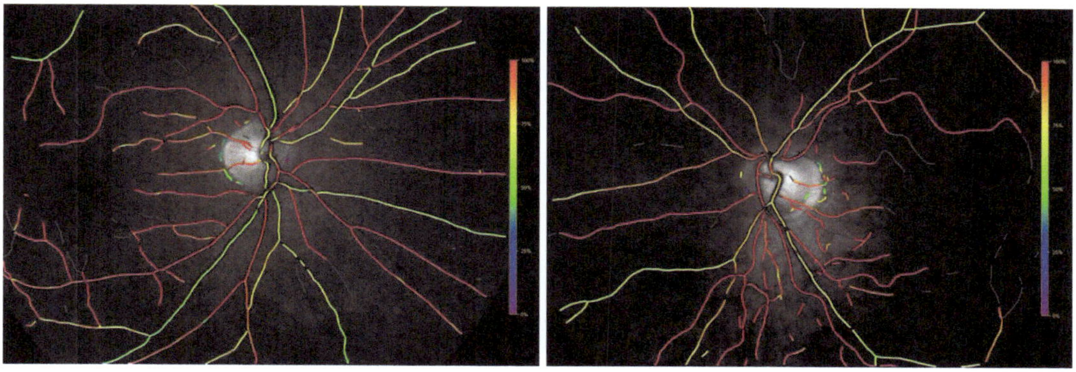

Fig. 8.8 Retinal vascular SO_2 maps shown in pseudocolor as generated by oximetry in a healthy (left) and glaucoma (right) subject. (Reprinted with permission from Olafsdottir et al., Ref. [236])

Oximetry has also been performed during light flicker stimulation, which serves as a physiological challenge to the retina. The ability of the retina to respond to this challenge can be used as a marker for neurovascular coupling. During light flicker stimulation, in response to increased metabolic demand, vasodilation and increased SO_{2V} have been established in healthy subjects [234, 235, 247–250]. However, the vascular response to light flicker stimulation has been shown to be impaired in glaucoma [251, 252]. Also, light flicker-induced changes in SO_{2V} and SO_{2AV} were shown to decrease in POAG [239]. In one study, light flicker-induced changes in SO_{2V} were not correlated with RNFL thickness, suggesting changes in the oxygen metabolic function precede structural changes in glaucoma [253].

Hyperspectral Oximetry

Hyperspectral oximetry is a technique in which reflectance images at several wavelengths are acquired quasi-simultaneously and analyzed to determine SO_2. In 2007, one of the earlier approaches employed white light to illuminate the retina and used multiple lenses paired with separate filters to isolate wavelengths of interest [254]. This technique generated images at 14 wavelengths but was time intensive and required an expensive large-format imaging camera. Another technique incorporated a liq-

uid crystal tunable filter into a commercial slit lamp biomicroscope to generate retinal images at 50 wavelengths [255]. However, this technique required up to 15 min for image acquisition and produced SO_{2V} values lower than expected. Also in 2007, a computer tomographic imaging spectrometer was introduced that was capable of rapid hyperspectral imaging using multiplexing, but was limited to small-field imaging [256]. More recently, a hyperspectral technique utilizing a tunable filter to generate retinal images at 27 wavelengths per second was developed [257]. Similar to dual wavelength oximetry, studies using hyperspectral oximetry also found increased SO_{2V} and decreased SO_{2AV} in glaucoma [258, 259]. Hyperspectral oximetry was also utilized to assess total hemoglobin content near the ONH, which may serve as a marker for glaucoma development [257, 260].

Multimodal Imaging

Despite recent advances in technology, no single imaging modality can provide comprehensive information about structural and functional changes necessary for diagnosis and monitoring of glaucoma. A common approach to overcome limitations is the use of multimodal imaging, wherein imaging technologies are combined or used nearly simultaneous to supplement the information provided from a single modality. One example of multimodal imaging in experimental research is the coupling of fluorescence and AOSLO imaging. Specifically, fluorescence AOSLO has been used to image the RGC and RPE in mice and macaques [261, 262]. AOSLO has also been used in combination with SD-OCT to generate 3D models of LC to study pore geometry [263]. In another study, AOSLO and 2PF were combined for imaging of photoreceptors, RGCs, and autofluorescence from the RPE in nonhuman primates [264]. Recently, a study combined AO with FLIM and 2PF to visualize RGCs and retinal capillaries in mice [265]. These multimodal imaging techniques may become applicable for studying human glaucoma in the future.

Retinal oximetry has been performed in combination with OCT imaging modalities to provide complementary information on retinal structure and function. Specifically, combined assessment of retinal vascular SO_2 and RNFL thickness measured by retinal tomography and OCT has been performed in glaucoma [237, 240]. The relationship between retinal vascular SO_2 and choroidal thickness has been reported [266]. Retrospective analysis of data from

multimodal images obtained in the Leuven Eye Study determined relationships between retinal vascular SO_2, blood flow, choroidal thickness, and ocular pulse amplitude [267]. Multimodal imaging has been employed to provide information about retinal metabolic function. Specifically, the rates of retinal oxygen delivery and metabolism have been reported in healthy, diabetic, and sickle cell retinopathy subjects based on measurements of SO_2 paired with blood flow from Doppler OCT [248, 268, 269]. Figure 8.9 depicts OCT, OCTA, and Doppler OCT imaging coupled with oximetry in the same human eye to assess retinal structure, capillary perfusion, and total retinal blood flow and derive rates of inner retinal oxygen delivery and metabolism (unpublished data). These metrics are useful to define retinal oxygen extraction fraction, which serves as an indicator of adequacy of the retinal circulation to meet the metabolic demand [234, 269]. Future application of these multimodal imaging techniques may potentially identify physiological biomarkers for detecting development and progression of glaucoma.

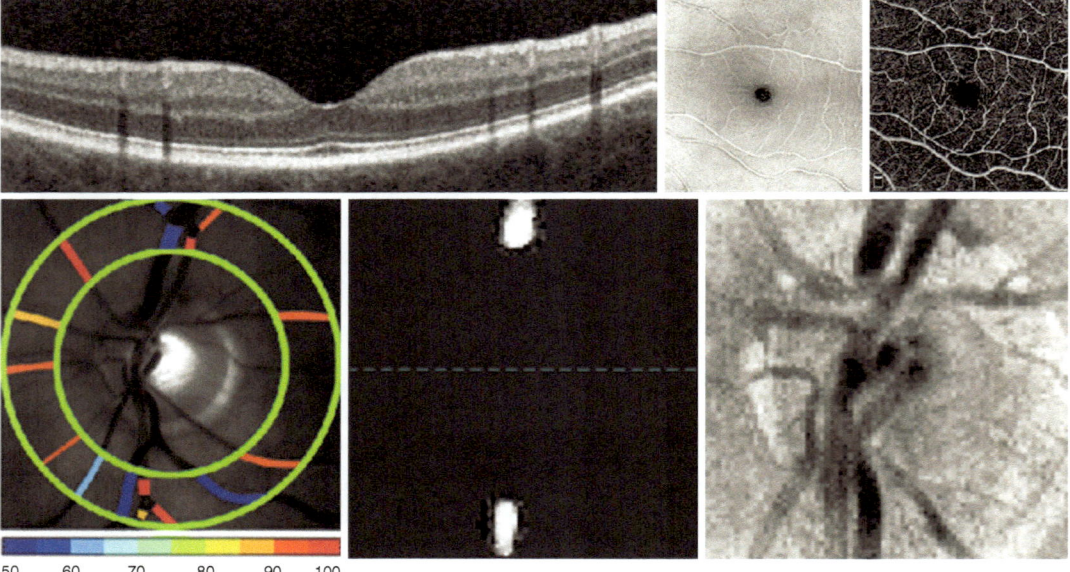

Fig. 8.9 Multimodal assessment of retinal thickness, microvascular perfusion, blood flow, vascular SO_2, and rates of oxygen delivery and metabolism by OCT, OCTA, Doppler OCT, and oximetry. (Images were obtained in the same eye)

Artificial Intelligence

Machine learning is a branch of artificial intelligence concerned with the development of algorithms or models for a computer to use and progressively improve at a given task. In glaucoma research, machine learning approaches have been applied to improve diagnostic accuracy of OCT image-based ONH structural parameters and classification of glaucoma [27, 270]. Also, numerical modeling has been applied to OCT images to estimate TM stiffness [271]. A machine-learning model for classification of glaucomatous ONH based on OCT and LSFG was developed, demonstrating the performance of neural network classifier [272]. Based on combined OCT and LSFG data, a neural network was trained and shown to be an identifier of disc parameters [273]. Deep learning (DL) is an advanced, sometimes automated class of machine learning used for diagnostic assessment of ocular diseases [274–278]. DL has been applied to retinal images obtained by various imaging modalities and shows promise for diagnostic screening and disease progression monitoring. Specifically, detection of photoreceptors was made possible by application of DL to AOSLO images [157, 279, 280]. Several studies reported DL applied to fundus images was capable of glaucoma diagnosis [281–286]. Furthermore, DL diagnosed the onset of glaucoma from macular OCT images and improved segmentation of ONH tissue using ONH OCT images [287, 288]. The challenging task of distinguishing glaucoma suspects from early glaucoma subjects was performed with the use of wide-field SS-OCT images processed by a DL technique [289]. Finally, applied to wide-field SLO images, DL was shown to detect VF defect severity [290]. Emerging novel computational techniques coupled with advancements in imaging technologies show great promise for screening and early detection of glaucoma prior to the onset of irreversible vision loss. In the future, it is conceivable multimodal imaging and artificial intelligence approaches will eventually become integrated into clinical practice and improve management of glaucoma.

Compliance with Ethical Requirements Mahnaz Shahidi and Anthony Felder declare that they have no conflict of interest. All procedures followed were in accordance with the ethical standards of the responsible committee on human experimentation (institutional and national) and with the Helsinki Declaration of 1975, as revised in 2000. Informed consent was obtained from all patients for being included in the study. No animal studies were carried out by the authors for this article.

References

1. Tham YC, Li X, Wong TY, Quigley HA, Aung T, Cheng CY. Global prevalence of glaucoma and projections of glaucoma burden through 2040: a systematic review and meta-analysis. Ophthalmology. 2014;121(11):2081–90.
2. Davis BM, Crawley L, Pahlitzsch M, Javaid F, Cordeiro MF. Glaucoma: the retina and beyond. Acta Neuropathol. 2016;132(6):807–26.
3. Fan N, Wang P, Tang L, Liu X. Ocular blood flow and normal tension glaucoma. Biomed Res Int. 2015;2015:308505.
4. Nakazawa T. Ocular blood flow and influencing factors for glaucoma. Asia-Pac J Ophthalmol (Philadelphia, Pa). 2016;5(1):38–44.
5. Promelle V, Daouk J, Bouzerar R, Jany B, Milazzo S, Baledent O. Ocular blood flow and cerebrospinal fluid pressure in glaucoma. Acta Radiologica Open. 2016;5(2):2058460115624275.
6. Gross J, Moore N, Do T, Huang A, Gama W, Siesky B, et al. Current imaging modalities for assessing ocular blood flow in glaucoma. Acta Ophthalmol. 2016;10(3):104–12.
7. Adhi M, Duker JS. Optical coherence tomography--current and future applications. Curr Opin Ophthalmol. 2013;24(3):213–21.
8. Fujimoto J, Swanson E. The development, commercialization, and impact of optical coherence tomography. Invest Ophthalmol Vis Sci. 2016;57(9):OCT1–OCT13.
9. Fujimoto JG, Pitris C, Boppart SA, Brezinski ME. Optical coherence tomography: an emerging technology for biomedical imaging and optical biopsy. Neoplasia. 2000;2(1–2):9–25.
10. Townsend KA, Wollstein G, Schuman JS. Imaging of the retinal nerve fibre layer for glaucoma. Br J Ophthalmol. 2009;93(2):139–43.
11. Huang D, Swanson EA, Lin CP, Schuman JS, Stinson WG, Chang W, et al. Optical coherence tomography. Science. 1991;254(5035):1178–81.
12. Swanson EA, Izatt JA, Hee MR, Huang D, Lin CP, Schuman JS, et al. In vivo retinal imaging by optical coherence tomography. Opt Lett. 1993;18(21):1864–6.
13. Fercher AF, Hitzenberger CK, Drexler W, Kamp G, Sattmann H. In vivo optical coherence tomography. Am J Ophthalmol. 1993;116(1):113–4.

14. Gabriele ML, Wollstein G, Ishikawa H, Kagemann L, Xu J, Folio LS, et al. Optical coherence tomography: history, current status, and laboratory work. Invest Ophthalmol Vis Sci. 2011;52(5):2425–36.

15. Lavinsky F, Wollstein G, Tauber J, Schuman JS. The future of imaging in detecting glaucoma progression. Ophthalmology. 2017;124(12s):S76–s82.

16. Mwanza JC, Budenz DL. New developments in optical coherence tomography imaging for glaucoma. Curr Opin Ophthalmol. 2018;29(2):121–9.

17. Cifuentes-Canorea P, Ruiz-Medrano J, Gutierrez-Bonet R, Pena-Garcia P, Saenz-Frances F, Garcia-Feijoo J, et al. Analysis of inner and outer retinal layers using spectral domain optical coherence tomography automated segmentation software in ocular hypertensive and glaucoma patients. PLoS One. 2018;13(4):e0196112.

18. Ghassibi MP, Chien JL, Patthanathamrongkasem T, Abumasmah RK, Rosman MS, Skaat A, et al. Glaucoma diagnostic capability of circumpapillary retinal nerve fiber layer thickness in circle scans with different diameters. J Glaucoma. 2017;26(4):335–42.

19. Khoueir Z, Jassim F, Poon LY, Tsikata E, Ben-David GS, Liu Y, et al. Diagnostic capability of peripapillary three-dimensional retinal nerve fiber layer volume for glaucoma using optical coherence tomography volume scans. Am J Ophthalmol. 2017;182:180–93.

20. Sharifipour F, Morales E, Lee JW, Giaconi J, Afifi AA, Yu F, et al. Vertical macular asymmetry measures derived from SD-OCT for detection of early glaucoma. Invest Ophthalmol Vis Sci. 2017;58(10):4310–7.

21. Mwanza JC, Budenz DL, Godfrey DG, Neelakantan A, Sayyad FE, Chang RT, et al. Diagnostic performance of optical coherence tomography ganglion cell--inner plexiform layer thickness measurements in early glaucoma. Ophthalmology. 2014;121(4):849–54.

22. Loewen NA, Zhang X, Tan O, Francis BA, Greenfield DS, Schuman JS, et al. Combining measurements from three anatomical areas for glaucoma diagnosis using Fourier-domain optical coherence tomography. Br J Ophthalmol. 2015;99(9):1224–9.

23. Elbendary AM, Abd El-Latef MH, Elsorogy HI, Enaam KM. Diagnostic accuracy of ganglion cell complex substructures in different stages of primary open-angle glaucoma. Can J Ophthalmol Journal canadien d'ophtalmologie. 2017;52(4):355–60.

24. Zhang X, Dastiridou A, Francis BA, Tan O, Varma R, Greenfield DS, et al. Comparison of glaucoma progression detection by optical coherence tomography and visual field. PLoS One. 2017;184:63–74.

25. Tatham AJ, Medeiros FA. Detecting structural progression in glaucoma with optical coherence tomography. Ophthalmology. 2017;124(12s):S57–s65.

26. Zhang X, Loewen N, Tan O, Greenfield DS, Schuman JS, Varma R, et al. Predicting development of glaucomatous visual field conversion using baseline Fourier-domain optical coherence tomography. Am J Ophthalmol. 2016;163:29–37.

27. Omodaka K, Kikawa T, Shiga Y, Tsuda S, Yokoyama Y, Sato H, et al. Usefulness of axonal tract-dependent OCT macular sectors for evaluating structural change in normal-tension glaucoma. PLoS One. 2017;12(10):e0185649.

28. Kim YK, Ha A, Na KI, Kim HJ, Jeoung JW, Park KH. Temporal relation between macular ganglion cell-inner plexiform layer loss and peripapillary retinal nerve Fiber layer loss in glaucoma. Ophthalmology. 2017;124(7):1056–64.

29. Reis AS, O'Leary N, Yang H, Sharpe GP, Nicolela MT, Burgoyne CF, et al. Influence of clinically invisible, but optical coherence tomography detected, optic disc margin anatomy on neuroretinal rim evaluation. Invest Ophthalmol Vis Sci. 2012;53(4):1852–60.

30. Yapp M, Rennie G, Hennessy MP, Kalloniatis M, Zangerl B. The impact of optic nerve and related characteristics on disc area measurements derived from different imaging techniques. PLoS One. 2018;13(1):e0190273.

31. Gardiner SK, Ren R, Yang H, Fortune B, Burgoyne CF, Demirel S. A method to estimate the amount of neuroretinal rim tissue in glaucoma: comparison with current methods for measuring rim area. Am J Ophthalmol. 2014;157(3):540–9.e1-2.

32. Chauhan BC, Burgoyne CF. From clinical examination of the optic disc to clinical assessment of the optic nerve head: a paradigm change. Am J Ophthalmol. 2013;156(2):218–27.e2.

33. Chauhan BC, O'Leary N, AlMobarak FA, Reis ASC, Yang H, Sharpe GP, et al. Enhanced detection of open-angle glaucoma with an anatomically accurate optical coherence tomography-derived neuroretinal rim parameter. Ophthalmology. 2013;120(3):535–43.

34. Enders P, Schaub F, Adler W, Hermann MM, Dietlein TS, Cursiefen C, et al. Bruch's membrane opening-based optical coherence tomography of the optic nerve head: a useful diagnostic tool to detect glaucoma in macrodiscs. Eye (Lond). 2018;32(2):314–23.

35. Park K, Kim J, Lee J. Reproducibility of Bruch membrane opening-minimum rim width measurements with spectral domain optical coherence tomography. J Glaucoma. 2017;26(11):1041–50.

36. Chauhan BC, Danthurebandara VM, Sharpe GP, Demirel S, Girkin CA, Mardin CY, et al. Bruch's membrane opening minimum rim width and retinal nerve fiber layer thickness in a normal white population: a multicenter study. Ophthalmology. 2015;122(9):1786–94.

37. Nakanishi H, Suda K, Yoshikawa M, Akagi T, Kameda T, Ikeda HO, et al. Association of Bruch's membrane opening and optic disc morphology to axial length and visual field defects in eyes with primary open-angle glaucoma. Graefes Arch Clin Exp Ophthalmol = Albrecht von Graefes Archiv fur klinische und experimentelle Ophthalmologie. 2018;256(3):599–610.

38. Han JC, Lee EJ, Kim SB, Kee C. The characteristics of deep optic nerve head morphology in myopic normal tension glaucoma. Invest Ophthalmol Vis Sci. 2017;58(5):2695–704.

39. Kim YW, Jeoung JW, Kim YK, Park KH. Clinical implications of in vivo Lamina Cribrosa imaging in glaucoma. Int J Mol Sci. 2017;26(9):753–61.

40. Shoji T. Correlation between Lamina Cribrosa tilt, myopia and glaucoma using optical coherence tomography with a wide band femtosecond mode-locked laser. Nippon Ganka Gakkai Zasshi. 2016;120(11):764–71.

41. Beotra MR, Wang X, Tun TA, Zhang L, Baskaran M, Aung T, et al. In vivo three-dimensional Lamina Cribrosa strains in healthy, ocular hypertensive, and Glaucoma eyes following acute intraocular pressure elevation. PLoS One. 2018;59(1):260–72.

42. Spaide RF, Koizumi H, Pozzoni MC. Enhanced depth imaging spectral-domain optical coherence tomography. Am J Ophthalmol. 2008;146(4):496–500.

43. Furlanetto RL, Vessani RM, Paranhos A Jr, Zhang X, Cole E, Pillar A, et al. The effect of change in intraocular pressure on choroidal structure in glaucomatous eyes. PLoS One. 2017;58(7):3278–85.

44. Lin Z, Huang S, Huang P, Guo L, Shen X, Zhong Y. The diagnostic use of choroidal thickness analysis and its correlation with visual field indices in glaucoma using spectral domain optical coherence tomography. PLoS One. 2017;12(12):e0189376.

45. Sacconi R, Deotto N, Merz T, Morbio R, Casati S, Marchini G. SD-OCT choroidal thickness in advanced primary open-angle glaucoma. J Glaucoma. 2017;26(6):523–7.

46. Akil H, Al-Sheikh M, Falavarjani KG, Francis B, Chopra V. Choroidal thickness and structural glaucoma parameters in glaucomatous, preperimetric glaucomatous, and healthy eyes using swept-source OCT. Eur J Ophthalmol. 2017;27(5):548–54.

47. Prata TS, Lopes FS, Prado VG, Almeida I, Matsubara I, Dorairaj S. In vivo analysis of glaucoma-related features within the optic nerve head using enhanced depth imaging optical coherence tomography. PLoS One. 2017;12(7):e0180128.

48. Park HL, Kim SI, Park CK. Influence of the lamina cribrosa on the rate of global and localized retinal nerve fiber layer thinning in open-angle glaucoma. Medicine. 2017;96(14):e6295.

49. Triolo G, Rabiolo A, Shemonski ND, Fard A, Di Matteo F, Sacconi R, et al. Optical coherence tomography angiography macular and peripapillary vessel perfusion density in healthy subjects, glaucoma suspects, and glaucoma patients. Invest Ophthalmol Vis Sci. 2017;58(13):5713–22.

50. Dastiridou A, Chopra V. Potential applications of optical coherence tomography angiography in glaucoma. Curr Opin Ophthalmol. 2018;29(3):226–33.

51. de Carlo TE, Romano A, Waheed NK, Duker JS. A review of optical coherence tomography angiography (OCTA). Int J Retina Vitreous. 2015;1:5.

52. Kashani AH, Chen CL, Gahm JK, Zheng F, Richter GM, Rosenfeld PJ, et al. Optical coherence tomography angiography: a comprehensive review of current methods and clinical applications. Prog Retin Eye Res. 2017;60:66–100.

53. Koustenis A Jr, Harris A, Gross J, Januleviciene I, Shah A, Siesky B. Optical coherence tomography angiography: an overview of the technology and an assessment of applications for clinical research. Br J Ophthalmol. 2017;101(1):16–20.

54. Wan KH, Leung CKS. Optical coherence tomography angiography in glaucoma: a mini-review. F1000Res. 2017;6:1686.

55. Akil H, Falavarjani KG, Sadda SR, Sadun AA. Optical coherence tomography angiography of the optic disc; an overview. J Ophthalmic Vis Res. 2017;12(1):98–105.

56. Rabiolo A, Gelormini F, Sacconi R, Cicinelli MV, Triolo G, Bettin P, et al. Comparison of methods to quantify macular and peripapillary vessel density in optical coherence tomography angiography. PLoS One. 2018;13(10):e0205773.

57. Pinhas A, Linderman R, Mo S, Krawitz BD, Geyman LS, Carroll J, et al. A method for age-matched OCT angiography deviation mapping in the assessment of disease- related changes to the radial peripapillary capillaries. PLoS One. 2018;13(5):e0197062.

58. Manalastas PIC, Zangwill LM, Daga FB, Christopher MA, Saunders LJ, Shoji T, et al. The association between macula and ONH optical coherence tomography angiography (OCT-A) vessel densities in glaucoma, glaucoma suspect, and healthy eyes. J Glaucoma. 2018;27(3):227–32.

59. Akil H, Huang AS, Francis BA, Sadda SR, Chopra V. Retinal vessel density from optical coherence tomography angiography to differentiate early glaucoma, pre-perimetric glaucoma and normal eyes. PLoS One. 2017;12(2):e0170476.

60. Geyman LS, Garg RA, Suwan Y, Trivedi V, Krawitz BD, Mo S, et al. Peripapillary perfused capillary density in primary open-angle glaucoma across disease stage: an optical coherence tomography angiography study. Br J Ophthalmol. 2017;101(9):1261–8.

61. Mammo Z, Heisler M, Balaratnasingam C, Lee S, Yu DY, Mackenzie P, et al. Quantitative optical coherence tomography angiography of radial peripapillary capillaries in glaucoma, glaucoma suspect, and normal eyes. Am J Ophthalmol. 2016;170:41–9.

62. Mo S, Phillips E, Krawitz BD, Garg R, Salim S, Geyman LS, et al. Visualization of radial Peripapillary capillaries using optical coherence tomography angiography: the effect of image averaging. PLoS One. 2017;12(1):e0169385.

63. Liu L, Jia Y, Takusagawa HL, Pechauer AD, Edmunds B, Lombardi L, et al. Optical coherence tomography angiography of the peripapillary retina in glaucoma. JAMA Ophthalmol. 2015;133(9):1045–52.

64. Suh MH, Zangwill LM, Manalastas PI, Belghith A, Yarmohammadi A, Medeiros FA, et al. Deep retinal layer microvasculature dropout detected by the optical coherence tomography angiography in glaucoma. Ophthalmology. 2016;123(12):2509–18.

65. Yarmohammadi A, Zangwill LM, Diniz-Filho A, Suh MH, Manalastas PI, Fatehee N, et al. Optical coherence tomography angiography vessel density in

healthy, glaucoma suspect, and glaucoma eyes. Invest Ophthalmol Vis Sci. 2016;57(9):OCT451–9.

66. Akagi T, Zangwill LM, Shoji T, Suh MH, Saunders LJ, Yarmohammadi A, et al. Optic disc microvasculature dropout in primary open-angle glaucoma measured with optical coherence tomography angiography. PLoS One. 2018;13(8):e0201729.

67. Hou H, Moghimi S, Zangwill LM, Shoji T, Ghahari E, Manalastas PIC, et al. Inter-eye asymmetry of optical coherence tomography angiography vessel density in bilateral glaucoma, glaucoma suspect, and healthy eyes. Am J Ophthalmol. 2018;190:69–77.

68. Shoji T, Zangwill LM, Akagi T, Saunders LJ, Yarmohammadi A, Manalastas PIC, et al. Progressive macula vessel density loss in primary open-angle glaucoma: a longitudinal study. Am J Ophthalmol. 2017;182:107–17.

69. Akagi T, Iida Y, Nakanishi H, Terada N, Morooka S, Yamada H, et al. Microvascular density in glaucomatous eyes with hemifield visual field defects: an optical coherence tomography angiography study. Am J Ophthalmol. 2016;168:237–49.

70. Chen CL, Bojikian KD, Wen JC, Zhang Q, Xin C, Mudumbai RC, et al. Peripapillary retinal nerve fiber layer vascular microcirculation in eyes with glaucoma and single-hemifield visual field loss. JAMA Ophthalmol. 2017;135(5):461–8.

71. Suh MH, Zangwill LM, Manalastas PI, Belghith A, Yarmohammadi A, Medeiros FA, et al. Optical coherence tomography angiography vessel density in glaucomatous eyes with focal Lamina Cribrosa defects. Ophthalmology. 2016;123(11):2309–17.

72. Yarmohammadi A, Zangwill LM, Diniz-Filho A, Suh MH, Yousefi S, Saunders LJ, et al. Relationship between optical coherence tomography angiography vessel density and severity of visual field loss in glaucoma. Ophthalmology. 2016;123(12):2498–508.

73. Yarmohammadi A, Zangwill LM, Diniz-Filho A, Saunders LJ, Suh MH, Wu Z, et al. Peripapillary and macular vessel density in patients with glaucoma and single-hemifield visual field defect. Ophthalmology. 2017;124(5):709–19.

74. Flammer J, Orgul S, Costa VP, Orzalesi N, Krieglstein GK, Serra LM, et al. The impact of ocular blood flow in glaucoma. Prog Retin Eye Res. 2002;21(4):359–93.

75. Mohindroo C, Ichhpujani P, Kumar S. Current imaging modalities for assessing ocular blood flow in glaucoma. J Curr Glaucoma Pract. 2016;10(3):104–12.

76. Harris A, Kagemann L, Ehrlich R, Rospigliosi C, Moore D, Siesky B. Measuring and interpreting ocular blood flow and metabolism in glaucoma. Can J Ophthalmol Journal canadien d'ophtalmologie. 2008;43(3):328–36.

77. Riva CE, Geiser M, Petrig BL, Beijing PRCOBFRA. Ocular blood flow assessment using continuous laser Doppler flowmetry. Acta Ophthalmol. 2010;88(6):622–9.

78. Resch H, Schmidl D, Popa-Cherecheanu A, Chua J, Garhofer G, Schmetterer L, et al. Comparative study of optical coherence tomography angiography and phase-resolved Doppler optical coherence tomography for measurement of retinal blood vessels caliber. Acta Ophthalmol. 2018;7(4):18.

79. Harris A. The effects of antioxidants on ocular blood flow in patients with glaucoma. Acta Ophthalmol. 2018;96(2):e237–e41.

80. Kurysheva NI, Parshunina OA, Shatalova EO, Kiseleva TN, Lagutin MB, Fomin AV. Value of structural and hemodynamic parameters for the early detection of primary open-angle glaucoma. Curr Eye Res. 2017;42(3):411–7.

81. Moore NA, Harris A, Wentz S, Verticchio Vercellin AC, Parekh P, Gross J, et al. Baseline retrobulbar blood flow is associated with both functional and structural glaucomatous progression after 4 years. Br J Ophthalmol. 2017;101(3):305–8.

82. Magureanu M, Stanila A, Bunescu LV, Armeanu C. Color Doppler imaging of the retrobulbar circulation in progressive glaucoma optic neuropathy. Rom J Ophthalmol. 2016;60(4):237–48.

83. Siesky B, Harris A, Carr J, Verticchio Vercellin A, Hussain RM, Parekh Hembree P, et al. Reductions in Retrobulbar and retinal capillary blood flow strongly correlate with changes in optic nerve head and retinal morphology over 4 years in open-angle glaucoma patients of African descent compared with patients of European descent. J Glaucoma. 2016;25(9):750–7.

84. Moore D, Harris A, Wudunn D, Kheradiya N, Siesky B. Dysfunctional regulation of ocular blood flow: a risk factor for glaucoma? Clin Ophthalmol (Auckland, NZ). 2008;2(4):849–61.

85. Leitgeb RA, Werkmeister RM, Blatter C, Schmetterer L. Doppler optical coherence tomography. Prog Retin Eye Res. 2014;41:26–43.

86. Wang Y, Bower BA, Izatt JA, Tan O, Huang D. In vivo total retinal blood flow measurement by Fourier domain Doppler optical coherence tomography. J Biomed Opt. 2007;12(4):041215.

87. Wang Y, Bower BA, Izatt JA, Tan O, Huang D. Retinal blood flow measurement by circumpapillary Fourier domain Doppler optical coherence tomography. J Biomed Opt. 2008;13(6):064003.

88. Singh AS, Kolbitsch C, Schmoll T, Leitgeb RA. Stable absolute flow estimation with Doppler OCT based on virtual circumpapillary scans. Biomed Opt Express. 2010;1(4):1047–58.

89. Wehbe H, Ruggeri M, Jiao S, Gregori G, Puliafito CA, Zhao W. Automatic retinal blood flow calculation using spectral domain optical coherence tomography. Opt Express. 2007;15(23):15193–206.

90. Dai C, Liu X, Zhang HF, Puliafito CA, Jiao S. Absolute retinal blood flow measurement with a dual-beam Doppler optical coherence tomography. Invest Ophthalmol Vis Sci. 2013;54(13):7998–8003.

91. Blatter C, Coquoz S, Grajciar B, Singh AS, Bonesi M, Werkmeister RM, et al. Dove prism based rotating dual beam bidirectional Doppler OCT. Biomed Opt Express. 2013;4(7):1188–203.

92. Doblhoff-Dier V, Schmetterer L, Vilser W, Garhofer G, Groschl M, Leitgeb RA, et al. Measurement of the total retinal blood flow using dual beam Fourier-domain Doppler optical coherence tomography with orthogonal detection planes. Biomed Opt Express. 2014;5(2):630–42.

93. Trasischker W, Werkmeister RM, Zotter S, Baumann B, Torzicky T, Pircher M, et al. In vitro and in vivo three-dimensional velocity vector measurement by three-beam spectral-domain Doppler optical coherence tomography. J Biomed Opt. 2013;18(11):116010.

94. Werkmeister RM, Dragostinoff N, Palkovits S, Told R, Boltz A, Leitgeb RA, et al. Measurement of absolute blood flow velocity and blood flow in the human retina by dual-beam bidirectional Doppler fourier-domain optical coherence tomography. Invest Ophthalmol Vis Sci. 2012;53(10):6062–71.

95. Werkmeister RM, Dragostinoff N, Pircher M, Gotzinger E, Hitzenberger CK, Leitgeb RA, et al. Bidirectional Doppler Fourier-domain optical coherence tomography for measurement of absolute flow velocities in human retinal vessels. Opt Lett. 2008;33(24):2967–9.

96. Sehi M, Goharian I, Konduru R, Tan O, Srinivas S, Sadda SR, et al. Retinal blood flow in glaucomatous eyes with single-hemifield damage. Ophthalmology. 2014;121(3):750–8.

97. Baumann B, Potsaid B, Kraus MF, Liu JJ, Huang D, Hornegger J, et al. Total retinal blood flow measurement with ultrahigh speed swept source/Fourier domain OCT. Biomed Opt Express. 2011;2(6):1539–52.

98. Choi W, Baumann B, Liu JJ, Clermont AC, Feener EP, Duker JS, et al. Measurement of pulsatile total blood flow in the human and rat retina with ultrahigh speed spectral/Fourier domain OCT. Biomed Opt Express. 2012;3(5):1047–61.

99. Srinivasan VJ, Adler DC, Chen Y, Gorczynska I, Huber R, Duker JS, et al. Ultrahigh-speed optical coherence tomography for three-dimensional and en face imaging of the retina and optic nerve head. Invest Ophthalmol Vis Sci. 2008;49(11):5103–10.

100. Lee B, Choi W, Liu JJ, Lu CD, Schuman JS, Wollstein G, et al. Cardiac-gated En Face Doppler measurement of retinal blood flow using swept-source optical coherence tomography at 100,000 axial scans per second. Invest Ophthalmol Vis Sci. 2015;56(4):2522–30.

101. Tan O, Liu G, Liang L, Gao SS, Pechauer AD, Jia Y, et al. En face Doppler total retinal blood flow measurement with 70 kHz spectral optical coherence tomography. J Biomed Opt. 2015; 20(6):066004.

102. Wang Y, Fawzi AA, Varma R, Sadun AA, Zhang X, Tan O, et al. Pilot study of optical coherence tomography measurement of retinal blood flow in retinal and optic nerve diseases. Invest Ophthalmol Vis Sci. 2011;52(2):840–5.

103. Briers JD, Fercher AF. Retinal blood-flow visualization by means of laser speckle photography. Invest Ophthalmol Vis Sci. 1982;22(2):255–9.

104. Sugiyama T, Araie M, Riva CE, Schmetterer L, Orgul S. Use of laser speckle flowgraphy in ocular blood flow research. Acta Ophthalmol. 2010;88(7):723–9.

105. Tamaki Y, Araie M, Kawamoto E, Eguchi S, Fujii H. Non-contact, two-dimensional measurement of tissue circulation in choroid and optic nerve head using laser speckle phenomenon. Exp Eye Res. 1995;60(4):373–83.

106. Tsuda S, Kunikata H, Shimura M, Aizawa N, Omodaka K, Shiga Y, et al. Pulse-waveform analysis of normal population using laser speckle flowgraphy. Curr Eye Res. 2014;39(12):1207–15.

107. Inoue-Yanagimachi M, Himori N, Sato K, Kokubun T, Asano T, Shiga Y, et al. Association between mitochondrial DNA damage and ocular blood flow in patients with glaucoma. Br J Ophthalmol. 2019;103(8):1060–65.

108. Kiyota N, Shiga Y, Suzuki S, Sato M, Takada N, Maekawa S, et al. The effect of systemic hyperoxia on optic nerve head blood flow in primary open-angle glaucoma patients. Invest Ophthalmol Vis Sci. 2017;58(7):3181–8.

109. Himori N, Kunikata H, Shiga Y, Omodaka K, Maruyama K, Takahashi H, et al. The association between systemic oxidative stress and ocular blood flow in patients with normal-tension glaucoma. Graefes Arch Clin Exp Ophthalmol = Albrecht von Graefes Archiv für klinische und experimentelle Ophthalmologie. 2016;254(2):333–41.

110. Anraku A, Ishida K, Enomoto N, Takagi S, Ito H, Takeyama A, et al. Association between optic nerve head microcirculation and macular ganglion cell complex thickness in eyes with untreated normal tension glaucoma and a hemifield defect. J Ophthalmol. 2017;2017:3608396.

111. Kiyota N, Kunikata H, Shiga Y, Omodaka K, Nakazawa T. Ocular microcirculation measurement with laser speckle flowgraphy and optical coherence tomography angiography in glaucoma. Acta Ophthalmol. 2018;96(4):e485–e92.

112. Mursch-Edlmayr AS, Luft N, Podkowinski D, Ring M, Schmetterer L, Bolz M. Laser speckle flowgraphy derived characteristics of optic nerve head perfusion in normal tension glaucoma and healthy individuals: a pilot study. Sci Rep. 2018;8(1):5343.

113. Shiga Y, Omodaka K, Kunikata H, Ryu M, Yokoyama Y, Tsuda S, et al. Waveform analysis of ocular blood flow and the early detection of normal tension glaucoma. Invest Ophthalmol Vis Sci. 2013;54(12):7699–706.

114. Moroi H, Anraku A, Ishida K, Tomita G. Factors related to a right-left difference in visual field defect in the eyes with untreated normal tension glaucoma. J Ophthalmol. 2018;2018:4595214.

115. Shiga Y, Aizawa N, Tsuda S, Yokoyama Y, Omodaka K, Kunikata H, et al. Preperimetric Glaucoma Prospective Study (PPGPS): predicting visual field progression with basal optic nerve head blood flow

in normotensive PPG eyes. Transl Vis Sci Technol. 2018;7(1):11.

116. Shiga Y, Kunikata H, Aizawa N, Kiyota N, Maiya Y, Yokoyama Y, et al. Optic nerve head blood flow, as measured by laser speckle flowgraphy, is significantly reduced in preperimetric glaucoma. Curr Eye Res. 2016;41(11):1447–53.

117. Loureiro MM, Vianna JR, Danthurebandara VM, Sharpe GP, Hutchison DM, Nicolela MT, et al. Visibility of optic nerve head structures with spectral-domain and swept-source optical coherence tomography. J Glaucoma. 2017;26(9):792–7.

118. Hong EH, Shin YU, Kang MH, Cho H, Seong M. Wide scan imaging with swept-source optical coherent tomography for glaucoma diagnosis. PLoS One. 2018;13(4):e0195040.

119. Lee WJ, Na KI, Kim YK, Jeoung JW, Park KH. Diagnostic ability of wide-field retinal nerve fiber layer maps using swept-source optical coherence tomography for detection of preperimetric and early perimetric glaucoma. J Glaucoma. 2017;26(6):577–85.

120. Miura N, Omodaka K, Kimura K, Matsumoto A, Kikawa T, Takahashi S, et al. Evaluation of retinal nerve fiber layer defect using wide-field en-face swept-source OCT images by applying the inner limiting membrane flattening. PLoS One. 2017;12(10):e0185573.

121. Wang B, Lucy KA, Schuman JS, Sigal IA, Bilonick RA, Lu C, et al. Tortuous pore path through the glaucomatous Lamina Cribrosa. Sci Rep. 2018;8(1):7281.

122. Wang B, Nevins JE, Nadler Z, Wollstein G, Ishikawa H, Bilonick RA, et al. In vivo lamina cribrosa microarchitecture in healthy and glaucomatous eyes as assessed by optical coherence tomography. Invest Ophthalmol Vis Sci. 2013;54(13):8270–4.

123. Wang B, Nevins JE, Nadler Z, Wollstein G, Ishikawa H, Bilonick RA, et al. Reproducibility of in-vivo OCT measured three-dimensional human lamina cribrosa microarchitecture. PLoS One. 2014;9(4):e95526.

124. Angmo D, Nongpiur ME, Sharma R, Sidhu T, Sihota R, Dada T. Clinical utility of anterior segment swept-source optical coherence tomography in glaucoma. Oman J Ophthalmol. 2016;9(1):3–10.

125. Akil H, Huang P, Chopra V, Francis B. Assessment of anterior segment measurements with swept source optical coherence tomography before and after ab interno trabeculotomy (Trabectome) surgery. J Ophthalmol. 2016;2016:4861837.

126. Akil H, Chopra V, Al-Sheikh M, Ghasemi Falavarjani K, Huang AS, Sadda SR, et al. Swept-source OCT angiography imaging of the macular capillary network in glaucoma. Br J Ophthalmol. 2018;102:515–19.

127. Kuehlewein L, Tepelus TC, An L, Durbin MK, Srinivas S, Sadda SR. Noninvasive visualization and analysis of the human parafoveal capillary network using swept source OCT optical microangiography. Invest Ophthalmol Vis Sci. 2015;56(6):3984–8.

128. Chen S, Shu X, Nesper PL, Liu W, Fawzi AA, Zhang HF. Retinal oximetry in humans using visible-light optical coherence tomography [invited]. Biomed Opt Express. 2017;8(3):1415–29.

129. Chong SP, Bernucci M, Radhakrishnan H, Srinivasan VJ. Structural and functional human retinal imaging with a fiber-based visible light OCT ophthalmoscope. Biomed Opt Express. 2017;8(1):323–37.

130. Shu X, Beckmann L, Zhang H. Visible-light optical coherence tomography: a review. J Biomed Opt. 2017;22(12):1–14.

131. Chong SP, Merkle CW, Leahy C, Radhakrishnan H, Srinivasan VJ. Quantitative microvascular hemoglobin mapping using visible light spectroscopic optical coherence tomography. Biomed Opt Express. 2015;6(4):1429–50.

132. Ju MJ, Huang C, Wahl DJ, Jian Y, Sarunic MV. Visible light sensorless adaptive optics for retinal structure and fluorescence imaging. Opt Lett. 2018;43(20):5162–5.

133. Song W, Zhou L, Zhang S, Ness S, Desai M, Yi J. Fiber-based visible and near infrared optical coherence tomography (vnOCT) enables quantitative elastic light scattering spectroscopy in human retina. Biomed Opt Express. 2018;9(7):3464–80.

134. Chong SP, Zhang T, Kho A, Bernucci MT, Dubra A, Srinivasan VJ. Ultrahigh resolution retinal imaging by visible light OCT with longitudinal achromatization. Biomed Opt Express. 2018;9(4):1477–91.

135. Yi J, Wei Q, Liu W, Backman V, Zhang HF. Visible-light optical coherence tomography for retinal oximetry. Opt Lett. 2013;38(11):1796–8.

136. Soetikno BT, Beckmann L, Zhang X, Fawzi AA, Zhang HF. Visible-light optical coherence tomography oximetry based on circumpapillary scan and graph-search segmentation. Biomed Opt Express. 2018;9(8):3640–52.

137. Nesper PL, Soetikno BT, Zhang HF, Fawzi AA. OCT angiography and visible-light OCT in diabetic retinopathy. Vis Res. 2017;139:191–203.

138. Shu X, Liu W, Duan L, Zhang HF. Spectroscopic Doppler analysis for visible-light optical coherence tomography. J Biomed Opt. 2017;22(12):1–8.

139. Hoyt WF, Frisen L, Newman NM. Fundoscopy of nerve fiber layer defects in glaucoma. Investig Ophthalmol. 1973;12(11):814–29.

140. Airaksinen PJ, Alanko HI. Effect of retinal nerve fibre loss on the optic nerve head configuration in early glaucoma. Graefes Arch Clin Exp Ophthalmol = Albrecht von Graefes Archiv fur klinische und experimentelle Ophthalmologie. 1983;220(4):193–6.

141. Webb RH, Hughes GW, Pomerantzeff O. Flying spot TV ophthalmoscope. Appl Opt. 1980;19(17):2991–7.

142. Webb RH, Hughes GW. Scanning laser ophthalmoscope. IEEE Trans Biomed Eng. 1981;28(7):488–92.

143. Webb RH, Hughes GW, Delori FC. Confocal scanning laser ophthalmoscope. Appl Opt. 1987;26(8):1492–9.

144. Weinreb RN, Dreher AW, Bille JF. Quantitative assessment of the optic nerve head with the laser tomographic scanner. Int Ophthalmol. 1989;13(1–2):25–9.

145. Dreher AW, Tso PC, Weinreb RN. Reproducibility of topographic measurements of the normal and glaucomatous optic nerve head with the laser tomographic scanner. Am J Ophthalmol. 1991;111(2):221–9.

146. Wollstein G, Garway-Heath DF, Hitchings RA. Identification of early glaucoma cases with the scanning laser ophthalmoscope. Ophthalmology. 1998;105(8):1557–63.

147. Roorda A, Romero-Borja F, Donnelly Iii W, Queener H, Hebert T, Campbell M. Adaptive optics scanning laser ophthalmoscopy. Opt Express. 2002;10(9):405–12.

148. Dreher AW, Bille JF, Weinreb RN. Active optical depth resolution improvement of the laser tomographic scanner. Appl Opt. 1989;28(4):804–8.

149. Liang J, Grimm B, Goelz S, Bille JF. Objective measurement of wave aberrations of the human eye with the use of a Hartmann-Shack wave-front sensor. J Opt Soc Am A Opt Image Sci Vis. 1994;11(7):1949–57.

150. Fernandez EJ, Iglesias I, Artal P. Closed-loop adaptive optics in the human eye. Opt Lett. 2001;26(10):746–8.

151. Fernandez EJ, Vabre L, Hermann B, Unterhuber A, Povazay B, Drexler W. Adaptive optics with a magnetic deformable mirror: applications in the human eye. Opt Express. 2006;14(20):8900–17.

152. Zhang Y, Poonja S, Roorda A. MEMS-based adaptive optics scanning laser ophthalmoscopy. Opt Lett. 2006;31(9):1268–70.

153. Chen DC, Jones SM, Silva DA, Olivier SS. High-resolution adaptive optics scanning laser ophthalmoscope with dual deformable mirrors. J Opt Soc Am A Opt Image Sci Vis. 2007;24(5):1305–12.

154. Manzanera S, Helmbrecht MA, Kempf CJ, Roorda A. MEMS segmented-based adaptive optics scanning laser ophthalmoscope. Biomed Opt Express. 2011;2(5):1204–17.

155. Abraham E, Cahyadi H, Brossard M, Degert J, Freysz E, Yasui T. Development of a wavefront sensor for terahertz pulses. Opt Express. 2016;24(5):5203–11.

156. Ferguson RD, Zhong Z, Hammer DX, Mujat M, Patel AH, Deng C, et al. Adaptive optics scanning laser ophthalmoscope with integrated wide-field retinal imaging and tracking. J Opt Soc Am A Opt Image Sci Vis. 2010;27(11):A265–77.

157. Davidson B, Kalitzeos A, Carroll J, Dubra A, Ourselin S, Michaelides M, et al. Automatic cone photoreceptor localisation in healthy and Stargardt afflicted retinas using deep learning. Sci Rep. 2018;8(1):7911.

158. Venkateswaran K, Roorda A, Romero-Borja F. Theoretical modeling and evaluation of the axial resolution of the adaptive optics scanning laser ophthalmoscope. J Biomed Opt. 2004;9(1):132–8.

159. Williams DR. Imaging single cells in the living retina. Vis Res. 2011;51(13):1379–96.

160. Chen MF, Chui TY, Alhadeff P, Rosen RB, Ritch R, Dubra A, et al. Adaptive optics imaging of healthy and abnormal regions of retinal nerve fiber bundles of patients with glaucoma. Invest Ophthalmol Vis Sci. 2015;56(1):674–81.

161. Hood DC, Lee D, Jarukasetphon R, Nunez J, Mavrommatis MA, Rosen RB, et al. Progression of local glaucomatous damage near fixation as seen with adaptive optics imaging. Transl Vis Sci Technol. 2017;6(4):6.

162. Huang G, Luo T, Gast TJ, Burns SA, Malinovsky VE, Swanson WH. Imaging glaucomatous damage across the temporal raphe. Invest Ophthalmol Vis Sci. 2015;56(6):3496–504.

163. Ivers KM, Li C, Patel N, Sredar N, Luo X, Queener H, et al. Reproducibility of measuring lamina cribrosa pore geometry in human and nonhuman primates with in vivo adaptive optics imaging. Invest Ophthalmol Vis Sci. 2011;52(8):5473–80.

164. Vilupuru AS, Rangaswamy NV, Frishman LJ, Smith EL 3rd, Harwerth RS, Roorda A. Adaptive optics scanning laser ophthalmoscopy for in vivo imaging of lamina cribrosa. J Opt Soc Am A Opt Image Sci Vis. 2007;24(5):1417–25.

165. Ivers KM, Sredar N, Patel NB, Rajagopalan L, Queener HM, Twa MD, et al. In Vivo Changes in Lamina Cribrosa Microarchitecture and Optic Nerve Head Structure in Early Experimental Glaucoma. PLoS ONE. 2015;10(7):e0134223.

166. Akagi T, Hangai M, Takayama K, Nonaka A, Ooto S, Yoshimura N. In vivo imaging of lamina cribrosa pores by adaptive optics scanning laser ophthalmoscopy. Invest Ophthalmol Vis Sci. 2012;53(7):4111–9.

167. Rossi EA, Granger CE, Sharma R, Yang Q, Saito K, Schwarz C, et al. Imaging individual neurons in the retinal ganglion cell layer of the living eye. Proc Natl Acad Sci U S A. 2017;114(3):586–91.

168. Miller DT, Williams DR, Morris GM, Liang J. Images of cone photoreceptors in the living human eye. Vis Res. 1996;36(8):1067–79.

169. Masella BD, Hunter JJ, Williams DR. Rod photopigment kinetics after photodisruption of the retinal pigment epithelium. Invest Ophthalmol Vis Sci. 2014;55(11):7535–44.

170. Hasegawa T, Ooto S, Takayama K, Makiyama Y, Akagi T, Ikeda HO, et al. Cone integrity in glaucoma: an adaptive-optics scanning laser ophthalmoscopy study. Am J Ophthalmol. 2016;171:53–66.

171. Nork TM, Ver Hoeve JN, Poulsen GL, Nickells RW, Davis MD, Weber AJ, et al. Swelling and loss of photoreceptors in chronic human and experimental glaucomas. Arch Ophthalmol. 2000;118(2):235–45.

172. Liang J, Williams DR, Miller DT. Supernormal vision and high-resolution retinal imaging through adaptive optics. J Opt Soc Am A Opt Image Sci Vis. 1997;14(11):2884–92.

173. Hofer H, Chen L, Yoon GY, Singer B, Yamauchi Y, Williams DR. Improvement in retinal image quality with dynamic correction of the eye's aberrations. Opt Express. 2001;8(11):631–43.

174. Chew AL, Sampson DM, Kashani I, Chen FK. Agreement in cone density derived from gaze-directed single images versus wide-field montage using adaptive optics flood illumination ophthalmoscopy. Transl Vis Sci Technol. 2017;6(6):9.

175. Zaleska-Zmijewska A, Piatkiewicz P, Smigielska B, Sokolowska-Oracz A, Wawrzyniak ZM, Romaniuk D, et al. Retinal photoreceptors and microvascular changes in Prediabetes measured with adaptive optics (rtx1): a case-control study. J Diabetes Res. 2017;2017:4174292.

176. Zaleska-Zmijewska A, Wawrzyniak ZM, Ulinska M, Szaflik J, Dabrowska A, Szaflik JP. Human photoreceptor cone density measured with adaptive optics technology (rtx1 device) in healthy eyes: standardization of measurements. Medicine. 2017;96(25):e7300.

177. Choi SS, Zawadzki RJ, Keltner JL, Werner JS. Changes in cellular structures revealed by ultrahigh resolution retinal imaging in optic neuropathies. Invest Ophthalmol Vis Sci. 2008;49(5):2103–19.

178. Choi SS, Zawadzki RJ, Lim MC, Brandt JD, Keltner JL, Doble N, et al. Evidence of outer retinal changes in glaucoma patients as revealed by ultrahigh-resolution in vivo retinal imaging. Br J Ophthalmol. 2011;95(1):131–41.

179. Werner JS, Keltner JL, Zawadzki RJ, Choi SS. Outer retinal abnormalities associated with inner retinal pathology in nonglaucomatous and glaucomatous optic neuropathies. Eye (Lond). 2011;25(3):279–89.

180. Zwillinger S, Paques M, Safran B, Baudouin C. In vivo characterization of lamina cribrosa pore morphology in primary open-angle glaucoma. J Fr Ophtalmol. 2016;39(3):265–71.

181. Zawadzki RJ, Jones SM, Olivier SS, Zhao M, Bower BA, Izatt JA, et al. Adaptive-optics optical coherence tomography for high-resolution and high-speed 3D retinal in vivo imaging. Opt Express. 2005;13(21):8532–46.

182. Fernandez EJ, Povazay B, Hermann B, Unterhuber A, Sattmann H, Prieto PM, et al. Three-dimensional adaptive optics ultrahigh-resolution optical coherence tomography using a liquid crystal spatial light modulator. Vis Res. 2005;45(28):3432–44.

183. Zhang Y, Rha J, Jonnal R, Miller D. Adaptive optics parallel spectral domain optical coherence tomography for imaging the living retina. Opt Express. 2005;13(12):4792–811.

184. Dong ZM, Wollstein G, Wang B, Schuman JS. Adaptive optics optical coherence tomography in glaucoma. Prog Retin Eye Res. 2017;57:76–88.

185. Fortune B. In vivo imaging methods to assess glaucomatous optic neuropathy. Exp Eye Res. 2015;141:139–53.

186. Miller DT, Kocaoglu OP, Wang Q, Lee S. Adaptive optics and the eye (super resolution OCT). Eye (Lond). 2011;25(3):321–30.

187. Kocaoglu OP, Cense B, Jonnal RS, Wang Q, Lee S, Gao W, et al. Imaging retinal nerve fiber bundles using optical coherence tomography with adaptive optics. Vis Res. 2011;51(16):1835–44.

188. Cense B, Koperda E, Brown JM, Kocaoglu OP, Gao W, Jonnal RS, et al. Volumetric retinal imaging with ultrahigh-resolution spectral-domain optical coherence tomography and adaptive optics using two broadband light sources. Opt Express. 2009;17(5):4095–111.

189. Nadler Z, Wang B, Schuman JS, Ferguson RD, Patel A, Hammer DX, et al. In vivo three-dimensional characterization of the healthy human lamina cribrosa with adaptive optics spectral-domain optical coherence tomography. Invest Ophthalmol Vis Sci. 2014;55(10):6459–66.

190. Kocaoglu OP, Ferguson RD, Jonnal RS, Liu Z, Wang Q, Hammer DX, et al. Adaptive optics optical coherence tomography with dynamic retinal tracking. Biomed Opt Express. 2014;5(7):2262–84.

191. Zawadzki RJ, Choi SS, Fuller AR, Evans JW, Hamann B, Werner JS. Cellular resolution volumetric in vivo retinal imaging with adaptive optics-optical coherence tomography. Opt Express. 2009;17(5):4084–94.

192. Werkmeister RM, Cherecheanu AP, Garhofer G, Schmidl D, Schmetterer L. Imaging of retinal ganglion cells in glaucoma: pitfalls and challenges. Cell Tissue Res. 2013;353(2):261–8.

193. Liu Z, Kurokawa K, Zhang F, Lee JJ, Miller DT. Imaging and quantifying ganglion cells and other transparent neurons in the living human retina. Proc Natl Acad Sci U S A. 2017;114(48):12803–8.

194. Smith CA, Vianna JR, Chauhan BC. Assessing retinal ganglion cell damage. Eye (Lond). 2017;31(2):209–17.

195. Thanos S, Indorf L, Naskar R. In vivo FM: using conventional fluorescence microscopy to monitor retinal neuronal death in vivo. Trends Neurosci. 2002;25(9):441–4.

196. Higashide T, Kawaguchi I, Ohkubo S, Takeda H, Sugiyama K. In vivo imaging and counting of rat retinal ganglion cells using a scanning laser ophthalmoscope. Invest Ophthalmol Vis Sci. 2006;47(7):2943–50.

197. Smith CA, Chauhan BC. Imaging retinal ganglion cells: enabling experimental technology for clinical application. Prog Retin Eye Res. 2015;44:1–14.

198. Kerr JN, Denk W. Imaging in vivo: watching the brain in action. Nat Rev Neurosci. 2008;9(3):195–205.

199. Palmer AE, Tsien RY. Measuring calcium signaling using genetically targetable fluorescent indicators. Nat Protoc. 2006;1(3):1057–65.

200. Lee JK, Lu S, Madhukar A. Real-time dynamics of Ca2+, caspase-3/7, and morphological changes in retinal ganglion cell apoptosis under elevated pressure. PLoS One. 2010;5(10):e13437.

201. Wen X, Cahill AL, Barta C, Thoreson WB, Nawy S. Elevated pressure increases ca(2+) influx through AMPA receptors in select populations of retinal ganglion cells. Front Cell Neurosci. 2018;12:162.

202. Chen Q, Cichon J, Wang W, Qiu L, Lee SJ, Campbell NR, et al. Imaging neural activity using Thy1-GCaMP transgenic mice. Neuron. 2012;76(2):297–308.

203. Yin L, Masella B, Dalkara D, Zhang J, Flannery JG, Schaffer DV, et al. Imaging light responses of foveal ganglion cells in the living macaque eye. J Neurosci. 2014;34(19):6596–605.

204. Grinvald A, Anglister L, Freeman JA, Hildesheim R, Manker A. Real-time optical imaging of naturally evoked electrical activity in intact frog brain. Nature. 1984;308(5962):848–50.

205. Maclaurin D, Venkatachalam V, Lee H, Cohen AE. Mechanism of voltage-sensitive fluorescence in a microbial rhodopsin. Proc Natl Acad Sci U S A. 2013;110(15):5939–44.

206. St-Pierre F, Chavarha M, Lin MZ. Designs and sensing mechanisms of genetically encoded fluorescent voltage indicators. Curr Opin Chem Biol. 2015;27:31–8.

207. Balendra SI, Normando EM, Bloom PA, Cordeiro MF. Advances in retinal ganglion cell imaging. Eye (Lond). 2015;29(10):1260–9.

208. Cordeiro MF, Guo L, Luong V, Harding G, Wang W, Jones HE, et al. Real-time imaging of single nerve cell apoptosis in retinal neurodegeneration. Proc Natl Acad Sci U S A. 2004;101(36):13352–6.

209. Yap ZL, Verma S, Lee YF, Ong C, Mohla A, Perera SA. Glaucoma related retinal oximetry: a technology update. Clin Ophthalmol (Auckland, NZ). 2018;12:79–84.

210. Cordeiro MF, Migdal C, Bloom P, Fitzke FW, Moss SE. Imaging apoptosis in the eye. Eye (Lond). 2011;25(5):545–53.

211. Yang E, Al-Mugheiry TS, Normando EM, Cordeiro MF. Real-time imaging of retinal cell apoptosis by confocal scanning laser ophthalmoscopy and its role in glaucoma. Front Neurol. 2018;9:338.

212. Lakowicz JR, Szmacinski H, Nowaczyk K, Berndt KW, Johnson M. Fluorescence lifetime imaging. Anal Biochem. 1992;202(2):316–30.

213. Sauer L, Andersen KM, Dysli C, Zinkernagel MS, Bernstein PS, Hammer M. Review of clinical approaches in fluorescence lifetime imaging ophthalmoscopy. J Biomed Opt. 2018;23(9):1–20.

214. Schweitzer D, Schenke S, Hammer M, Schweitzer F, Jentsch S, Birckner E, et al. Towards metabolic mapping of the human retina. Microsc Res Tech. 2007;70(5):410–9.

215. Ramm L, Jentsch S, Augsten R, Hammer M. Fluorescence lifetime imaging ophthalmoscopy in glaucoma. Graefes Arch Clin Exp Ophthalmol = Albrecht von Graefes Archiv fur klinische und experimentelle Ophthalmologie. 2014;252(12):2025–6.

216. Johnson AW, Ammar DA, Kahook MY. Two-photon imaging of the mouse eye. Invest Ophthalmol Vis Sci. 2011;52(7):4098–105.

217. Zhang X, Liu N, Mak PU, Pun SH, Vai MI, Masihzadeh O, et al. Three-dimensional segmentation and quantitative measurement of the aqueous outflow system of intact mouse eyes based on spectral two-photon microscopy techniques. Invest Ophthalmol Vis Sci. 2016;57(7):3159–67.

218. Gonzalez JM Jr, Ko MK, Masedunskas A, Hong YK, Weigert R, Tan JCH. Toward in vivo two-photon analysis of mouse aqueous outflow structure and function. Exp Eye Res. 2017;158:161–70.

219. Nguyen C, Midgett D, Kimball EC, Steinhart MR, Nguyen TD, Pease ME, et al. Measuring deformation in the mouse optic nerve head and peripapillary sclera. Invest Ophthalmol Vis Sci. 2017;58(2):721–33.

220. Miura Y. Two-Photon Microscopy (TPM) and Fluorescence Lifetime Imaging Microscopy (FLIM) of Retinal Pigment Epithelium (RPE) of mice in vivo. Methods Mol Biol. 2018;1753:73–88.

221. Aptel F, Olivier N, Deniset-Besseau A, Legeais JM, Plamann K, Schanne-Klein MC, et al. Multimodal nonlinear imaging of the human cornea. Invest Ophthalmol Vis Sci. 2010;51(5):2459–65.

222. Chu ER, Gonzalez JM Jr, Tan JC. Tissue-based imaging model of human trabecular meshwork. J Ocul Pharmacol Ther. 2014;30(2–3):191–201.

223. Huang AS, Gonzalez JM Jr, Le PV, Heur M, Tan JC. Sources of structural autofluorescence in the human trabecular meshwork. Invest Ophthalmol Vis Sci. 2013;54(7):4813–20.

224. Tan JC, Gonzalez JM Jr, Hamm-Alvarez S, Song J. In situ autofluorescence visualization of human trabecular meshwork structure. Invest Ophthalmol Vis Sci. 2012;53(4):2080–8.

225. Gonzalez JM Jr, Heur M, Tan JC. Two-photon immunofluorescence characterization of the trabecular meshwork in situ. Invest Ophthalmol Vis Sci. 2012;53(7):3395–404.

226. Masihzadeh O, Ammar DA, Lei TC, Gibson EA, Kahook MY. Real-time measurements of nicotinamide adenine dinucleotide in live human trabecular meshwork cells: effects of acute oxidative stress. Exp Eye Res. 2011;93(3):316–20.

227. Lei Y, Garrahan N, Hermann B, Becker DL, Hernandez MR, Boulton ME, et al. Quantification of retinal transneuronal degeneration in human glaucoma: a novel multiphoton-DAPI approach. Invest Ophthalmol Vis Sci. 2008;49(5):1940–5.

228. Zijlstra WG, Buursma A, Meeuwsen-van der Roest WP. Absorption spectra of human fetal and adult oxyhemoglobin, de-oxyhemoglobin, carboxyhemoglobin, and methemoglobin. Clin Chem. 1991;37(9):1633–8.

229. Hammer M, Vilser W, Riemer T, Schweitzer D. Retinal vessel oximetry-calibration, compensation for vessel diameter and fundus pigmentation, and reproducibility. J Biomed Opt. 2008;13(5):054015.

230. Beach J. Pathway to retinal oximetry. Transl Vis Sci Technol. 2014;3(5):2.

231. Beach JM, Schwenzer KJ, Srinivas S, Kim D, Tiedeman JS. Oximetry of retinal vessels by dual-

wavelength imaging: calibration and influence of pigmentation. J Appl Physiol. 1999;86(2):748–58.

232. Hickam JB, Frayser R, Ross JC. A study of retinal venous blood oxygen saturation in human subjects by photographic means. Circulation. 1963;27:375–85.

233. Hardarson SH. Retinal oximetry. Acta Ophthalmol. 2013;91 Thesis 2:1–47.

234. Felder AE, Wanek J, Blair NP, Shahidi M. Inner retinal oxygen extraction fraction in response to light flicker stimulation in humans. Invest Ophthalmol Vis Sci. 2015;56(11):6633–7.

235. Garhofer G, Bek T, Boehm AG, Gherghel D, Grunwald J, Jeppesen P, et al. Use of the retinal vessel analyzer in ocular blood flow research. Acta Ophthalmol. 2010;88(7):717–22.

236. Olafsdottir OB, Vandewalle E, Abegao Pinto L, Geirsdottir A, De Clerck E, Stalmans P, et al. Retinal oxygen metabolism in healthy subjects and glaucoma patients. Br J Ophthalmol. 2014;98(3):329–33.

237. Vandewalle E, Abegao Pinto L, Olafsdottir OB, De Clerck E, Stalmans P, Van Calster J, et al. Oximetry in glaucoma: correlation of metabolic change with structural and functional damage. Acta Ophthalmol. 2014;92(2):105–10.

238. Olafsdottir OB, Hardarson SH, Gottfredsdottir MS, Harris A, Stefansson E. Retinal oximetry in primary open-angle glaucoma. Invest Ophthalmol Vis Sci. 2011;52(9):6409–13.

239. Ramm L, Jentsch S, Peters S, Augsten R, Hammer M. Investigation of blood flow regulation and oxygen saturation of the retinal vessels in primary open-angle glaucoma. Graefe's archive for clinical and experimental ophthalmology = Albrecht von Graefes Archiv fur klinische und experimentelle. Fortschr Ophthalmol. 2014;252(11):1803–10.

240. Hammer M, Ramm L, Agci T, Augsten R. Venous retinal oxygen saturation is independent from nerve fibre layer thickness in glaucoma patients. Acta Ophthalmol. 2016;94(3):e243–4.

241. Mitchell P, Leung H, Wang JJ, Rochtchina E, Lee AJ, Wong TY, et al. Retinal vessel diameter and open-angle glaucoma: the Blue Mountains eye study. Ophthalmology. 2005;112(2):245–50.

242. Rao A, Agarwal K, Mudunuri H, Padhy D, Roy AK, Mukherjee S. Vessel caliber in normal tension and primary open angle glaucoma eyes with Hemifield damage. J Glaucoma. 2017;26(1):46–53.

243. Shin YU, Lee SE, Cho H, Kang MH, Seong M. Analysis of Peripapillary retinal vessel diameter in unilateral normal-tension glaucoma. J Ophthalmol. 2017;2017:8519878.

244. Yap ZL, Ong C, Lee YF, Tsai A, Cheng C, Nongpiur ME, et al. Retinal oximetry in subjects with glaucomatous hemifield asymmetry. J Glaucoma. 2017;26(4):367–72.

245. Chang M, Yoo C, Kim SW, Kim YY. Retinal vessel diameter, retinal nerve fiber layer thickness, and intraocular pressure in korean patients with normal-tension glaucoma. Am J Ophthalmol. 2011;151(1):100–5 e1.

246. Kim JM, Sae Kim M, Ju Jang H, Ho Park K, Caprioli J. The association between retinal vessel diameter and retinal nerve fiber layer thickness in asymmetric normal tension glaucoma patients. Invest Ophthalmol Vis Sci. 2012;53(9):5609–14.

247. Felder AE, Wanek J, Blair NP, Shahidi M. Retinal vascular and oxygen temporal dynamic responses to light flicker in humans. Invest Ophthalmol Vis Sci. 2017;58(13):5666–72.

248. Palkovits S, Lasta M, Told R, Schmidl D, Werkmeister R, Cherecheanu AP, et al. Relation of retinal blood flow and retinal oxygen extraction during stimulation with diffuse luminance flicker. Sci Rep. 2015;5:18291.

249. Garhofer G, Zawinka C, Resch H, Huemer KH, Dorner GT, Schmetterer L. Diffuse luminance flicker increases blood flow in major retinal arteries and veins. Vis Res. 2004;44(8):833–8.

250. Formaz F, Riva CE, Geiser M. Diffuse luminance flicker increases retinal vessel diameter in humans. Curr Eye Res. 1997;16(12):1252–7.

251. Garhofer G, Zawinka C, Resch H, Huemer KH, Schmetterer L, Dorner GT. Response of retinal vessel diameters to flicker stimulation in patients with early open angle glaucoma. J Glaucoma. 2004;13(4):340–4.

252. Riva CE, Salgarello T, Logean E, Colotto A, Galan EM, Falsini B. Flicker-evoked response measured at the optic disc rim is reduced in ocular hypertension and early glaucoma. Invest Ophthalmol Vis Sci. 2004;45(10):3662–8.

253. Hammer M, Ramm L, Peters S, Augsten R. Is the change of oxygen extraction from retinal vessels upon flicker light stimulation dependent on the nerve fiber layer thickness in glaucoma patients? Graefe's archive for clinical and experimental ophthalmology = Albrecht von Graefes Archiv fur klinische und experimentelle. Fortschr Ophthalmol. 2016;254(8):1649–50.

254. Ramella-Roman JC, Mathews SA. Spectroscopic measurements of oxygen saturation in the retina. IEEE J Sel Top Quant Electron. 2007;13(6):1697–703.

255. Mordant DJ, Al-Abboud I, Muyo G, Gorman A, Sallam A, Ritchie P, et al. Spectral imaging of the retina. Eye (Lond). 2011;25(3):309–20.

256. Johnson WR, Wilson DW, Fink W, Humayun M, Bearman G. Snapshot hyperspectral imaging in ophthalmology. J Biomed Opt. 2007;12(1):014036.

257. Desjardins M, Sylvestre JP, Jafari R, Kulasekara S, Rose K, Trussart R, et al. Preliminary investigation of multispectral retinal tissue oximetry mapping using a hyperspectral retinal camera. Exp Eye Res. 2016;146:330–40.

258. Shahidi AM, Hudson C, Tayyari F, Flanagan JG. Retinal oxygen saturation in patients with primary open-angle glaucoma using a non-flash hypespectral camera. Curr Eye Res. 2017;42(4):557–61.

259. Mordant DJ, Al-Abboud I, Muyo G, Gorman A, Harvey AR, McNaught AI. Oxygen saturation measurements of the retinal vasculature in

treated asymmetrical primary open-angle glaucoma using hyperspectral imaging. Eye (Lond). 2014;28(10):1190–200.

260. Gonzalez de la Rosa M, Gonzalez-Hernandez M, Sigut J, Alayon S, Radcliffe N, Mendez-Hernandez C, et al. Measuring hemoglobin levels in the optic nerve head: comparisons with other structural and functional parameters of glaucoma. Invest Ophthalmol Vis Sci. 2013;54(1):482–9.

261. Geng Y, Dubra A, Yin L, Merigan WH, Sharma R, Libby RT, et al. Adaptive optics retinal imaging in the living mouse eye. Biomed Opt Express. 2012;3(4):715–34.

262. Morgan JI, Hunter JJ, Masella B, Wolfe R, Gray DC, Merigan WH, et al. Light-induced retinal changes observed with high-resolution autofluorescence imaging of the retinal pigment epithelium. Invest Ophthalmol Vis Sci. 2008;49(8):3715–29.

263. Sredar N, Ivers KM, Queener HM, Zouridakis G, Porter J. 3D modeling to characterize lamina cribrosa surface and pore geometries using in vivo images from normal and glaucomatous eyes. Biomed Opt Express. 2013;4(7):1153–65.

264. Sharma R, Williams DR, Palczewska G, Palczewski K, Hunter JJ. Two-photon autofluorescence imaging reveals cellular structures throughout the retina of the living primate eye. Invest Ophthalmol Vis Sci. 2016;57(2):632–46.

265. Feeks JA, Hunter JJ. Adaptive optics two-photon excited fluorescence lifetime imaging ophthalmoscopy of exogenous fluorophores in mice. Biomed Opt Express. 2017;8(5):2483–95.

266. Van Keer K, Abegao Pinto L, Willekens K, Stalmans I, Vandewalle E. Correlation between peripapillary choroidal thickness and retinal vessel oxygen saturation in young healthy individuals and glaucoma patients. Invest Ophthalmol Vis Sci. 2015;56(6):3758–62.

267. Barbosa-Breda J, Van Keer K, Abegao-Pinto L. Improved discrimination between normal-tension and primary open-angle glaucoma with advanced vascular examinations - the Leuven eye study. Acta Ophthalmol. 2018;97:e50.

268. Palkovits S, Lasta M, Told R, Schmidl D, Boltz A, Napora KJ, et al. Retinal oxygen metabolism during normoxia and hyperoxia in healthy subjects. Invest Ophthalmol Vis Sci. 2014;55(8):4707–13.

269. Shahidi M, Felder AE, Tan O, Blair NP, Huang D. Retinal oxygen delivery and metabolism in healthy and sickle cell retinopathy subjects. Invest Ophthalmol Vis Sci. 2018;59(5):1905–9.

270. Miri MS, Abramoff MD, Kwon YH, Sonka M, Garvin MK. A machine-learning graph-based approach for 3D segmentation of Bruch's membrane opening from glaucomatous SD-OCT volumes. Med Image Anal. 2017;39:206–17.

271. Wang K, Johnstone MA, Xin C, Song S, Padilla S, Vranka JA, et al. Estimating human trabecular meshwork stiffness by numerical modeling and advanced OCT imaging. PLoS One. 2017;58(11):4809–17.

272. An G, Omodaka K, Tsuda S, Shiga Y, Takada N, Kikawa T, et al. Comparison of machine-learning classification models for glaucoma management. J Health Care Eng. 2018;2018:6874765.

273. Omodaka K, An G, Tsuda S, Shiga Y, Takada N, Kikawa T, et al. Classification of optic disc shape in glaucoma using machine learning based on quantified ocular parameters. PLoS One. 2017;12(12):e0190012.

274. Grewal PS, Oloumi F, Rubin U, Tennant MTS. Deep learning in ophthalmology: a review. Can J Ophthalmol Journal canadien d'ophtalmologie. 2018;53(4):309–13.

275. Matsuura M, Murata H, Asaoka R, Du XL, Li WB, Hu BJ. Application of artificial intelligence in ophthalmology. Sci Rep. 2018;11(9):1555–61.

276. Rahimy E. Deep learning applications in ophthalmology. Curr Opin Ophthalmol. 2018;29(3):254–60.

277. Ting DSW, Pasquale LR, Peng L, Campbell JP, Lee AY, Raman R, et al. Artificial intelligence and deep learning in ophthalmology. Br J Ophthalmol. 2018;103:167.

278. Hagiwara Y, Koh JEW, Tan JH, Bhandary SV, Laude A, Ciaccio EJ, et al. Computer-aided diagnosis of glaucoma using fundus images: a review. Comput Methods Prog Biomed. 2018;165:1–12.

279. Cunefare D, Fang L, Cooper RF, Dubra A, Carroll J, Farsiu S. Open source software for automatic detection of cone photoreceptors in adaptive optics ophthalmoscopy using convolutional neural networks. Sci Rep. 2017;7(1):6620.

280. Cunefare D, Langlo CS, Patterson EJ, Blau S, Dubra A, Carroll J, et al. Deep learning based detection of cone photoreceptors with multimodal adaptive optics scanning light ophthalmoscope images of achromatopsia. Biomed Opt Express. 2018;9(8):3740–56.

281. Ahn JM, Kim S, Ahn KS, Cho SH, Lee KB, Kim US. A deep learning model for the detection of both advanced and early glaucoma using fundus photography. PLoS One. 2018;13(11):e0207982.

282. Christopher M, Belghith A, Bowd C, Proudfoot JA, Goldbaum MH, Weinreb RN, et al. Performance of deep learning architectures and transfer learning for detecting glaucomatous optic neuropathy in fundus photographs. Sci Rep. 2018;8(1):16685.

283. Fu H, Cheng J, Xu Y, Zhang C, Wong DWK, Liu J, et al. Disc-aware ensemble network for glaucoma screening from fundus image. IEEE Trans Med Imaging. 2018;37(11):2493–501.

284. Jiang Y, Xia H, Xu Y, Cheng J, Fu H, Duan L, et al. Optic disc and cup segmentation with blood vessel removal from fundus images for glaucoma detection. PLoS One. 2018;2018:862–5.

285. Mitra A, Banerjee PS, Roy S, Roy S, Setua SK. The region of interest localization for glaucoma analysis from retinal fundus image using deep learning. Comput Methods Prog Biomed. 2018;165:25–35.

286. Shibata N, Tanito M, Mitsuhashi K, Fujino Y. Development of a deep residual learning algo-

rithm to screen for glaucoma from fundus photography. Sci Rep. 2018;8(1):14665.

287. Asaoka R, Murata H, Hirasawa K, Fujino Y, Matsuura M, Miki A, et al. Using deep learning and transform learning to accurately diagnose early-onset glaucoma from macular optical coherence tomography images. Am J Ophthalmol. 2018;198:136.

288. Devalla SK, Renukanand PK, Sreedhar BK, Subramanian G, Zhang L, Perera S, et al. DRUNET: a dilated-residual U-net deep learning network to segment optic nerve head tissues in optical coher-

ence tomography images. Biomed Opt Express. 2018;9(7):3244–65.

289. Muhammad H, Fuchs TJ, De Cuir N, De Moraes CG, Blumberg DM, Liebmann JM, et al. Hybrid deep learning on single wide-field optical coherence tomography scans accurately classifies Glaucoma suspects. J Glaucoma. 2017;26(12):1086–94.

290. Masumoto H, Tabuchi H, Nakakura S, Ishitobi N, Miki M, Enno H. Deep-learning classifier with an Ultrawide-field scanning laser ophthalmoscope detects Glaucoma visual field severity. J Glaucoma. 2018;27(7):647–52.

Correction to: Advances in Ocular Imaging in Glaucoma

Rohit Varma, Benjamin Y. Xu, Grace M. Richter, and Alena Reznik

---

Correction to:
R. Varma et al. (eds.), *Advances in Ocular Imaging in Glaucoma*, Essentials in Ophthalmology,
https://doi.org/10.1007/978-3-030-43847-0

The book was inadvertently published with incorrect affiliation of Rohit Varma in copyright page. His affiliation has now been amended to "Southern California Eye Institute, CHA Hollywood Presbyterian Medical Center, Los Angeles, CA, USA".

The updated version of this book can be found at
https://doi.org/10.1007/978-3-030-43847-0

© Springer Nature Switzerland AG 2020
R. Varma et al. (eds.), *Advances in Ocular Imaging in Glaucoma*, Essentials in Ophthalmology,
https://doi.org/10.1007/978-3-030-43847-0_9

Index

© Springer Nature Switzerland AG 2020
R. Varma et al. (eds.), *Advances in Ocular Imaging in Glaucoma*, Essentials in Ophthalmology,
https://doi.org/10.1007/978-3-030-43847-0